D. DEFOSSE

AF678665

BORRELIA

BORRELIA

STRAINS, VECTORS, HUMAN AND ANIMAL BORRELIOSIS

By

OSCAR FELSENFELD, M.Sc., M.D.,

Chief, Division of Communicable Diseases
Delta Regional Primate Research Center
Professor of Tropical Medicine and International Health
Tulane University School of Public Health and Tropical Medicine
Visiting Professor of Microbiology
Tulane University School of Medicine
Member, International Taxonomic
Subcommittee on Spirochaetales

WARREN H. GREEN, INC.
St. Louis, Missouri, U.S.A.

Published by

WARREN H. GREEN, INC.
10 South Brentwood Blvd.
St. Louis, Missouri 63105, U.S.A.

All rights reserved

© 1971, by WARREN H. GREEN, INC.

Library of Congress Catalog Card Number 72-127355

Printed in the United States of America
1-B (186)

DEDICATION

TO: Dr. M. Baltazard, Director Emeritus, Pasteur Institute, Teheran; Professor A. Rafyi, Director Emeritus, Hessarak Institute, Iran; Professor A. Geigy, Swiss Institute of Tropical Medicine, Basel; Dr. Charles M. Wheeler, Research Entomologist

and the Memory of the late Professor E. Brumpt, Parasitology Institute, Paris

whose patient instructions, friendly guidance, kind encouragement, competent support, and understanding criticism have made my studies of *Borrelia* possible and pleasurable during the past 35 years.

PREFACE

DESPITE PERIODIC REPORTS that tick-borne relapsing fever occurs sporadically over more than half the area of the entire Continental United States, the numerous deaths due to this disease in the drier parts of Asia and Africa including the thousands who become its victims in Ethiopia and the Sudan every year, the unknown toll in lives and suffering that the disease is still taking in Central and South America, and the ever-present danger of recurrence of epidemics should the louse-borne form burst out of its present confines if or when a disaster creates favorable conditions for such spread, only scanty notes on relapsing fever can be found in the medical literature of the United States today.

One is amazed at the confused nomenclature and the mass of misinformation concerning the transmission and vectors (some of which has managed to creep into even respectable textbooks). The considerable variations in the clinical picture during various outbreaks and in widely separated localities, and the unusual immunologic conditions that accompany the infection should be emphasized so that the medical profession can be alerted should an outbreak occur in this country.

The genus *Borrelia* that causes human relapsing fever includes some species that are of interest to the dentist *(Borrelia vincentii),* and to the veterinarian *(B. anserina, B. theileri). Borrelia* infections appear in man as relapsing fever and in animals as so-called fowl spirochetosis, or tick-transmitted spirochetosis in cattle, which are clinically defined entities. This monograph deals principally with human relapsing fever and fowl spirochetosis, while exploring other conditions in which borreliae may play a role. The discussion of the borreliae and their vectors, the pathology caused by them, and other features will be presented in separate chapters discussing borreliosis as human relapsing fever, cattle and fowl disease, and Vincent's angina, respectively. Each of these chapters will deal separately with the species of *Borrelia* involved, and with the consequences of the infection. Borreliae that have been isolated from vectors only, and not from man or animals, will also be enumerated.

O. F.

ACKNOWLEDGMENTS

THIS MONOGRAPH COULD NEVER HAVE GONE TO PRESS without the unselfish aid, help, and support of two persons. One of them, Dr. Addine G. Erskine, spent innumerable hours correcting, retyping, editing, proof-reading, and indexing this volume. Busy as she was as Director of the Gradwohl School of Laboratory Technique and with numerous professional organizations, other editorial tasks, and ranching (unfortunately or fortunately, no *B. theileri* has been isolated from her stock), she has always found time to cooperate on my writing ventures, including this monograph. I am sincerely and deeply indebted to her for all her most valuable help.

The other, Dr. W. Burgdorfer, Senior Medical Entomologist of the U.S.P.H.S. Rocky Mountain Laboratories, has never hesitated to replenish my stock of *Ornithodoros* whenever my "tickorium" went out of gear. I am very much grateful to him for all support he has so kindly furnished during the years, in addition to admiring his elegant experiments and publications.

Dr. W. E. Greer, Director of Animal Resources, Gulf South Research Institute, New Iberia, La., kindly checked the chapters on animal borreliosis. Most of the entomological statements which appeared 5 years ago were reviewed by Prof. G. Anastos, University of Maryland, and Prof. A. Rafyi at that time.

I am much obligated and sincerely grateful to Dr. A. D. M. Bryceson and his colleagues for permitting me to read and to quote their outstanding clinical study of relapsing fever in Ethiopia before publication, and to Dr. H. Hoogstraal for his encouragement.

Dr. T. C. Orihel, Adj. Professor of Parasitology, Tulane University, spent much valuable time and great effort providing me with and photographing arthropods for this book. His assistant, Mrs. B. van Duym, furnished several excellent drawings. Mrs. W. Martin of the Medical Illustration Service of this Center made additional valuable graphs. Dr. C. Jones, Smithsonian Institute, kindly selected and put at my disposal his photographs of Southeast African huts and rodent burrows. Dr. Jones also corrected and rectified the names of the mammals.

Dr. M. N. Wilderman, D.D.S., M.S., Professor and Head, Department of Periodontology, Louisiana University School of Dentistry, kindly furnished the photographs of Vincent's disease.

Mrs. M. LaCroix and Mrs. C. Bennett typed and retyped the numerous drafts as well as the final copy of the manuscript. Their diligence and help are appreciated greatly.

O. F.

CONTENTS

BORRELIA

I

HUMAN BORRELIOSIS (RELAPSING FEVER)

RELAPSING FEVER (borreliosis) may appear either in louse-borne epidemics or in sporadic tick-borne instances. The disease is characterized by recurring attacks of fever, usually of decreasing intensity and duration. Relapsing fever, however, may be of sufficient intensity as to terminate in death.

The disease has been named "febris recurrens," "recurrent fever," "famine fever," "spirillum fever," "spirochetal fever," "vagabond fever" (Spain), "fowl nest fever" (China), "gharib gez" (Iran), "Giesinger's bilious typhoid" (Egypt), "carapata" (Africa), "kim-putu," "gorgoya" (South America), "tick fever." It has also been given other *epitheton ornans* -es taken from local picturesque descriptive designations and from more or less fortunate combinations of greco-neo-latin terms. The generally accepted name, however, is relapsing fever and, in countries adhering to Latin nomenclature, "febris recurrens."

The causative agent, *Borrelia,* is insect-borne and is transferred from man to man directly only under unusual circumstances. The disease acquires epidemiologic importance principally among people who are compelled to live under unfavorable hygienic conditions. The epidemiologic aspects of endemic or tick-borne relapsing fever that is carried by some species of *Ornithodoros* depend upon the interrelationship of man and ticks, and often also on a mammalian host. There are challenging features and many little known aspects of this disease. The widespread relapsing fever outbreaks that developed during the end of and after World War II, the constant occurrence of the infection in Africa and Asia, and the apparent hitherto confused picture of vectors and agents in Central and South America have not as yet stimulated many researchers

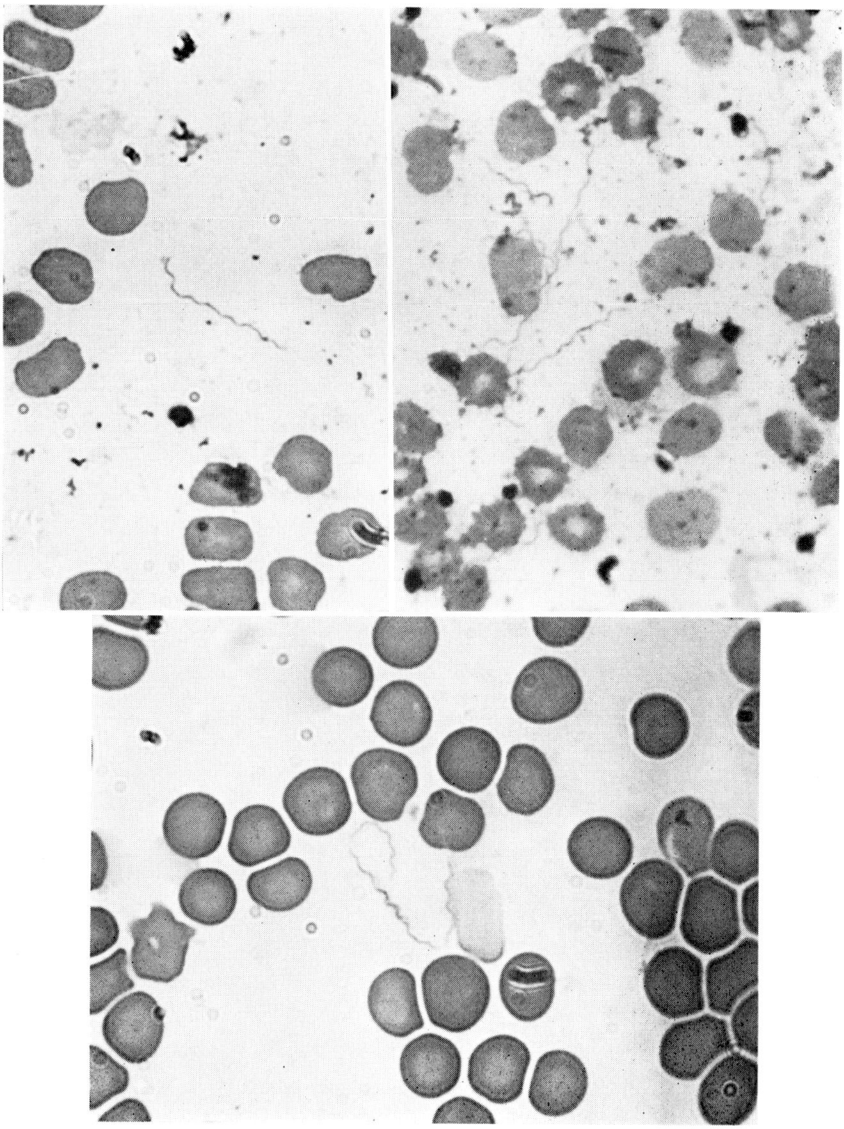

FIGURE 1. *Borrelia* in blood. Giemsa stain. x 950.

to delve into this problem. Neither have some interesting observations made during and after World War II fully penetrated into the world literature. While important basic research on *Borrelia* and its vectors is being performed in several institutions, the influence of the host-parasite relationship on the epidemiology of relapsing fever and the course of the disease in individual patients are stressed only in a few textbooks. It seemed desirable, therefore, to survey the literature on these aspects of relapsing fever, and to present such knowledge in a critical review which may assist scientists who wish to approach this manifold problem.

Several chapters in textbooks and review articles deal with more than one aspect of relapsing fever, as those of Hindle (363, 364, 365), Mühlens (509), Walters (709), Simmons (647), Geigy and Herbig (308), Mooser (500), Felsenfeld (264), Whitmore (731, 732), the Symposium on Relapsing Fever in the Americas in 1942, sponsored by the American Association for the Advancement of Science, and others. Geigy (303) summarized his long experience with relapsing fever in Africa, and Southern and Sanford (659) recently surveyed pertinent data on relapsing fever. Other reviews, dealing with specific problems of borreliosis, will be noted in the respective chapters.

HISTORY

Many historical accounts of relapsing fever are based on the studies of Scott (634).

Epidemic relapsing fever was recorded and described by Hippocrates in Thasos as "ardent fever" (308, 634). Bryceson *et al.* (127) believe that the "yellow fever" experienced in Europe during the VIth century may have been relapsing fever. The five epidemics of "sweating sickness" that swept England between 1485 and 1551 included outbreaks of relapsing fever (127, 491). Louse-borne typhus also prevailed at that time and "famine fever" was the common designation of both infections. Gloucestershire was wiped out in the beginning of the XVIIIth century by "famine fever." England and Ireland suffered from this disease also in the XVIIth and XVIIIth centuries. The first well-documented epidemic of relapsing fever was described in Ireland between 1739 and 1741 when Rutty recorded its clinical features. The epidemic then spread from Ireland to Scotland and England. The outbreak in 1834-1848 in Edinburg was particularly severe. The designation "relapsing fever" was first used by Craigie in 1843.

The Scandinavian countries became infected in 1788 from Russian ships that made port in Sweden. The last epidemic in Germany occurred from 1867 to 1868, in Ireland from 1868 to 1871. Later, improving hygienic conditions kept the disease from West Europe.

Louse-borne relapsing fever was imported into the United States from England and in 1844 caused the famous Philadelphia epidemic. This infection persisted in the eastern region of the United States for about 30 years. In 1874, there was a similar outbreak among Chinese laborers in California (193). Tick-borne relapsing fever was recognized soon after the West was settled (727).

The causative agent of epidemic relapsing fever was discovered in 1868 by Obermeier who did not publish his paper on this subject, however, until 1873 (507). This organism is now designated as *Borrelia recurrentis*. In the past, it was called *Spirocheta obermeieri, Protomycetum recurrentis, Spirocheta recurrentis,* and other names (128).

Little is known about louse-borne relapsing fever before the XVIIIth century except that it prevailed in cold and poor countries where lice were common. It was known to have occurred in Africa and in China (149, 363, 641).

Carlisle (145), Geigy (303), and others agree that Livingstone was the first to note in 1857 that tick-borne relapsing fever was present in Angola and Mozambique and that the disease was familiar to the local African and Portuguese inhabitants. Lamoureaux (430) reported that Drury had observed tick-borne relapsing fever during his trip to Madagascar in 1702-1720 but it remained for Cook (198) in Uganda to notice the presence of *Borrelia* in the blood. Ross and Milne (613) in the same area and simultaneously Dutton and Todd (250) in the Congoes, as well as Koch (417) in East Africa, confirmed these findings and demonstrated that tick-borne *Borrelia* may cause disease in monkeys and man. Both Dutton and Todd contracted the disease, and Dutton died of it (303).

The "bilious typhoid" in Egypt, described by Griesinger in 1857 (617) appears to have been relapsing fever, but Napoleon's surgeons were the first to diagnose relapsing fever correctly in that country (395).

Among other investigations of historical importance are those of Koch (418) in East Africa which resulted in the naming of a *Borrelia* strain *Spirochaeta kochi;* the studies of Novy and Knapp (547) of the movement of *B. recurrentis,* and their observation that antibodies begin to develop during the first attack of the disease; the review of Hindle (361) of relapsing fever in tropical Africa; the investigation of the mode of division of borreliae and a review of the *Borrelia* problem by Dobell (243); the experiments of Ross (612) on patas monkeys with strains isolated in Uganda; the survey of the distribution of the vector *(Ornithodoros moubata)* of *B. duttonii* in Africa by Nuttall (548); the attempts of Nicolle *et al.* (536) to transmit tick-borne borreliae to lice; the first demonstration of the infectiousness of the coxal fluid of *O. moubata* by Todd (684); and the study of the ecology of *O. moubata* between 1892 to 1905 by Todd (685) which led him to predict that as travel increased, the tick, and with it also tick-borne relapsing fever, would spread further through Africa.

Relapsing fever has been observed in all parts of the world, except Australia, New Zealand, and Oceania, where only solitary imported cases have been seen (363).

In Africa, reports of past occurrences are available from the former Gold Coast (617, 618). LeGac (439) described an epidemic in Oudaii (Chad) between 1925-1928. Hawkins (338) studied *B. duttonii* infections in Tanganyika. Fendall and Grounds (269) believed the disease to be retreating in Kenya, where louse-borne relapsing fever was introduced by refugees from Abyssinia (296). The Sudan had several louse-borne outbreaks. After the first world war, repatriates brought infected lice with them to that country. The ensuing epidemic stopped only at the forest (439). Atkey (30) described this 1926-1928 outbreak. Kirk (411) believed that the constant population movement from and to Abyssinia steadily supplies the Sudan with infected lice. Hindle (365) observed that louse-borne relapsing fever swept over the major part of the northern part of Africa during 1925-1928.

Relapsing fever is not new to many parts of Africa. Kirk (411) noted the louse-borne relapsing fever was introduced into the Sudan from Egypt between 1908 and 1924, in 1926 from French West Africa, and during the Abyssinian War in 1936 from Italian Africa.

Egypt suffered during the Napoleonic invasion (see above) and, according to Kamal *et al.* (395), experienced an outbreak that was recognized as relapsing fever by Sandwirth and Engel in 1884. The disease has been systematically studied since 1906 in that country.

Algeria, Tunisia, and Morocco have been recording louse-borne relapsing fever since 1903 (534, 535, 641, 642). The 1907-1914 epidemic in Algeria offered an occasion for numerous scientific studies.

Somaliland, closely adjacent to the Abyssinian-Sudanese focus of relapsing fever, experienced tick-borne cases among troops in her formerly British territory (244). Other occurrences of the disease were recorded by Italian authors (610). Moise (497) commented on relapsing fever in Somaliland, pointing out that the most effective African tick vector, *O. moubata,* is very scarce in that area. He suspected that there were other transmitting agents. A similar dispute arose in Madagascar, where Lamoureaux (430) recorded the appearance of the disease in military personnel who used the route between Morandava and Majuna in 1911 and 1912. Suldey (672) encountered tick-borne cases on the west coast of Madagascar in spite of the scarcity of a recognized vector.

In South Africa, relapsing fever remained undiagnosed until an outbreak was observed in the Cape Province among miners who had come from the North and had brought with them the tick *O. moubata* as a good-luck charm which then began to thrive in their huts.

In Yemen, in Asia Minor, Franchini (277) was unable to find ticks that were capable of conveying borreliae and concluded that the louse was the only vector.

During the first world war, Egypt was heavily hit by louse-borne relapsing fever (395, 670). In the four years between 1916 and 1920, 40,000 cases were recorded. Syria and Turkey also became infested (628, 734). Mesopotamia had an outbreak in 1918 among Turkish railroad workers (519). During the aftermath of World War I, from February to August 1920, troops became infected in Birjand, East Persia. Relapsing fever in the absence of lice was reported in Jinnuk, East Persia (337, 739), while the areas of Sharifabad, Meshed, and Turbad had ticks as well as human lice that were able to carry borreliae.

In India, where Mackie was the first to state in 1907 that the human louse carried epidemic relapsing fever, numerous episodes of the disease were recorded. "Spirillar fever" was described in a group of Ghurka tea garden workers in Darjeeling (392). Roy (614) reported an outbreak in the Seoni District (Upper Provinces) in 1919-1920. It was believed (206, 207) that louse-borne relapsing fever was endemic in Agra and Oudh, and spread from there to other areas. Gill (316) published the statistics on the outbreaks in the Punjab in 1869, 1878, 1891, 1906, and 1920 which claimed 26,000 lives.

Browse (114) described tick-borne recurrent fever in Qetta, principally among military camp followers who were new to the area and who lacked immunity.

Cases were described in Afghanistan by Avanessov (33) who did not, however, find the vector.

China has been the home of louse-borne relapsing fever for a long time. Records in the western literature are available from West China (387), Sechuan (388), an outbreak in an oprhanage in Peiping (172), and a review of 337 cases treated in the Peiping University Medical College Hospital between 1921-1937 (176). Toyoda (687) studied *Borrelia* strains collected in Manchuria.

Indochina was infected from China. There were 373 cases in Hanoi during the first half of 1912 (508). The disease was found in Nghê-An (357). Casoux (149) and Millous (495) described the course of relapsing fever that during the 1910-1911 cool period alone took about 500 lives in Annam. The disease spilled over into Thailand (733). Further data are not available from that country.

As stated previously, louse-borne relapsing fever came from China to the United States in 1874 (494). Later, however, tick-borne relapsing fever was the type of the disease that prevailed on the Pacific Coast. A summary of such instances for the years 1921-1937 was presented by Wheeler (737). Meador (489) reported 5 cases from Colorado. Bannister (66), Hemingway *et al.* (356) and Thayer (680) rendered further reports from the Southwest and Northwest. Graham (321) described a case of a boy who entered a cave in Denton County, Texas, that has been known for years to harbor infested ticks, and became ill with relapsing fever. Kemp *et al.* (408) surveyed the epidemiology in Texas. Closson (183) described it in Kansas. Briggs (111) and Coleman (193, 194) reviewed the situation in California. Palmer and Crawford (560) reported an outbreak in British Columbia. The transmitting tick was not found in that episode in Canada.

Louse-borne relapsing fever was observed in Panama by Connor (197). Tick-borne cases were seen in March and April, 1921, in hunters and in rats captured in the Arraiján area (68). Dunn and Clark (248) studied animal hosts and vectors in Panama.

Relapsing fever was introduced to Ecuador probably from Colombia during the revolution in 1896 (443). It is now tick-borne in both countries.

Chiriboga (164) reported louse-borne infections from Peru. Prado (588, 589) described the history of the disease in that country, dating back to population movements in the late XIXth century.

During the Balkan War louse-borne relapsing fever was not common in Macedonia in spite of the presence of the vector. The disease was at home in the trenches of World War I, principally in the countries of the Central Powers and in East Europe. An outbreak initiated by the distribution of Austrian prisoners of war in Serbia for work in the fields lasted 6 months (377). Cantacuzène (143) noted that louse-borne relapsing fever was endemic in the eastern part (Besarabia) of Rumania but there was an upsurge of the disease and of epidemic typhus in 1916. Poland was heavily infested at that time. The city of Lodz alone had 343 cases between March and December, 1917 (473). Sterling-Okunewski (669) and Lipinski (453) reported additional instances in Poland and in Hungary. Oettinger and Helbreich (551) related the course of the disease on the Russian front.

The tick-borne form has been observed in the Caucasus since 1928 by Maruashvilli (475) and in Tashkent (398). A thorough analysis of the natural foci of the disease in Turkemenia followed later by Petrishcheva (571).

It appears that the association of man and louse that was considered a somewhat vexing event but not an evil part of life, until hygienic concepts began to prevail in the 19th and 20th centuries, has endowed the history of louse-borne relapsing fever with a continuity that has been interrupted by epidemic outbursts perhaps only at times when the immunity of larger population groups reached a low ebb, or when hitherto uninfected populations came into contact with infected groups of people.

Louse-borne relapsing fever spread during and after World War I over large areas of the Old World as a result of the propagation of lice among dislocated soldiers and civilians living under unhygienic conditions, who were compelled to move about from locale to locale. These epidemics gave impetus to the study of the disease. Most basic clinical and epidemiologic concepts of relapsing fever were elaborated during these periods. Further outbreaks, as well as less extensive epidemics, have also been studied thoroughly and will be analyzed in subsequent chapters. Among these belongs the recognition of the continuity and contiguity of louse-borne relapsing fever.

The study of tick-borne or endemic borreliosis went through the same phase as the rest of microbiology, when the major interest apparently was to discover new species and strains. Borreliosis is a dynamic condition, a cyclic disease characterized by a cyclic causative agent. No wonder that great numbers of species have been proposed on the basis of minor or not fully understood strain variations and mutations, incomplete knowledge of the vector, and epidemiologic observations that were not extended far enough "longitudinally" and "laterally." Some of the taxonomy both of *Borrelia* and *Ornithodoros* still has to be untangled, principally in Central Asia and South America. A further complication arises from the transliteration of the names of some authors, principally in the U.S.S.R., who had published in Russian and German, choosing the method of transcription of certain letters of the Cyrillic alphabet more or less arbitrarily. One encounters in the literature Pavlovsky, Pawlowski, Pavlovskii, Pavlovskyi; *B. latishevyi, B. latischewyi, B. latishewyi,* and so forth. The Reader is asked for his kind indulgence when encountering such discrepancies, principally in the references.

CAUSATIVE AGENT

Taxonomy

Detailed discussions of the taxonomy and biology of *Borrelia* have been presented by Baltazard *et. al.* (62), Davis (222, 223),

Dobell (243), Geigy (303), Geigy and Herbig (308), Geiman (314), Gelman (315), Heisch (342, 343), Hindle (363, 364, 365), Johnstone (386), Moursund (507), Nicolle and Anderson (521, 526), Schuhardt (630), Walters (709), and others.

The common *Borrelia* strains that cause relapsing fever in man are listed in Table 1, together with their vectors and geographic distribution.

The genus *Borrelia* Swellengrebel 1907 is a member of the family Treponemataceae Robinson 1948 which belongs in the order Spirochaetales Buchanan 1918. Until recent electron microscopic

TABLE 1
BORRELIAE CAUSING HUMAN RELAPSING FEVER, THEIR VECTORS AND GEOGRAPHICAL DISTRIBUTION

Borrelia	*Vector*	*Geographical Distribution*
B. recurrentis	*Pediculus humanus*	Potentially cosmopolitan
B. hispanica	*Ornithodoros erraticus erraticus*	Mediterranean, Middle East, East and West Africa, from Uganda to Iran
crocidurae group*	*O. erraticus sonrai*	
B. crocidurae		Middle East, Central Africa
B. microti		Middle East
B. merionesi		West Africa
B. dipodilli		East Africa
B. duttonii	*O. moubata*	Principally East and South Africa
B. persica	*O. tholozani* (O. papillipes)	Eastern Mediterranean, Arab Peninsula, Iran, Central Asia
B. latyschewii	*O. tartakovskyi*	Central Asia
B. caucasica	*O. verrucosus*	Caucasus
B. venezolensis	*O. rudis* (O.venezolensis)	Northern part of South America
unnamed (dugesii?)	*O. talaje*	Central and South America, Western US, Canada
B. mazzottii	*O. talaje* (substrain?)	Central, possibly also South Amercia, Texas
B. turicatae	*O. turicata*	Central and South America, Western US, Canada
B. parkerii	*O. parkeri*	Western US, Canada
B. hermsii	*O. hermsi*	Western US

* Human pathogenicity low.

and some biochemical studies were completed, members of the genus *Borrelia* were described merely as unicellular, spiral organisms without a rigid cell wall, with broad and irregular, loose spirals of inconstant amplitude, motile by an axial filament, easily stained with aniline dyes but difficult to cultivate on artificial media, parasitic to man and animals, and principally propagated by insects (102, 132).

Borreliae have been designated by a number of different names in the past, such as *Protomycetum, Spirochaeta, Spirocheta, Spirillum, Spironema, Treponema* etc. The European literature, including that of the U.S.S.R., still uses *Spirochaeta* in certain publications whereas this term should be reserved only for free-living forms.

The identification of *Borrelia* species according to the usual bacteriologic characteristics is difficult if not impossible. The organisms are not easily cultured, and their antigenic phase variations during relapses, which is one of the principal features of the agent, often preclude serologic diagnosis. Animal responses may be variable. The morphologic characteristics of all recognized species are about the same (128, 132) and often depend on the fixative and staining method employed (46, 47, 196 and others). This is particularly true when silver impregnation methods are used (386). Other means of classification had to be sought and were found in the agent-vector relationship.

B. recurrentis, the cause of epidemic relapsing fever, was originally designated *Protomycetum recurrentis* by Lebert in 1874; *Spirochaeta obermeieri* by Cohn in 1875; and *Treponema recurrentis* by Schaudinn in 1905, before it was classified as a member of the genus *Borrelia.* Some of its sub-strains will be discussed later.

The primarily tick-borne borreliae have been classified by Geigy (303) as *B. duttonii* Novy and Knapp 1906, the agent of East African relapsing fever or African tick fever; *B. hispanica* de Buen 1926, the cause of Hispano-African relapsing fever; *B. duttonii* var. *crocidurae* Leger 1917 (synonymous with *B. crocidurae, B. merionesi,* and *B. microti*) and *B. dipodilli* Heisch 1950 as members of the "crocidurae" subgroup; *B. persica* Dschunkowsky 1913 as the cause of Asiatic relapsing fever; *B. turicatae* Brumpt 1933, *B. parkerii* Davis 1942, and *B. hermsii* Davis 1942, the agents of the disease in the United States; *B. venezolensis* Brumpt 1921, the cause of South American infections. This classification takes into account disease, geographical distribution, natural vectors, and animal reservoirs (if known). The names of the borreliae are closely linked with those of their vectors, principally because agent-vector specificity is very strong in borreliae (118, 223, 386). *B. recurrentis* is propagated by the body louse *Pediculus humanus* Linnaeus 1758, the other species by *Ornithodoros* ticks. These relationships will be discussed in detail later.

Davis (219, 220) called attention to difficulties in studying the specificity of strain-vector-host relationships. Some experimenters study the organism by injecting borreliae or crushed insects; others feed the vectors on infected animals. It is quite possible that different technics give divergent results. After extensive studies Baltazard (50) agreed with the concept of tick-specificity of borreliae, principally in the United States. The recent investigation of 2623 *O. canestrini* by Skrynnik (650) also tends to confirm this concept. We assume, therefore, that *B. duttonii* is harbored by *Ornithodoros moubata, B. hispanica* by *O. erraticus erraticus,* the "crocidurae" subgroup by *O. erraticus sonrai, B. persica* by *O. tholozani (=O. papillipes), B. turicatae* by *O. turicata, B. parkerii* by *O. parkeri, B. hermsii* by *O. hermsi, B. venezolensis* by *O. rudis (=O. venezuelensis),* while the vector relationship of *B. mazzottii* is not yet settled.

In laboratory experiments it may happen that a tick is used in transmission studies and that such a tick is already carrying a different strain of the same *Borrelia* or another *Borrelia.* Studies with wild ticks, therefore, always have to be evaluated carefully. In well controlled experiments, however, some unusual *Borrelia*-tick relationships have been observed. For instance Brumpt (117) found transmission of *B. crocidurae* by *O. moubata* and *O. marocanus.* Davis and Burgdorfer (226) isolated a strain of *B. parkerii* in Oregon which was transmitted not only by *O. parkeri* but also by *O. turicata.* Davies (222) listed further exceptions. Brumpt (122), a firm believer in the unitarian acarine concept, invited attention to possible mutations of the borreliae in the host that may influence the outcome of such studies. Walters (709) and Felsenfeld (264) believed that *Borrelia*-tick species specificity follows the rules closely but is not always exact. Walton (713) went one step further by investigating the feeding habits of ticks and reached the conclusion that many acarines have a strong preference for a single mammalian host.

Nicolle and Anderson (521) believed that borreliae were originally parasites of small rodents and were later transferred by ticks to man and from man to lice. Thus, ticks conserve and lice propagate these organisms. They are systemic parasites of argasid ticks and lice according to Burgdorfer (129). Baker and Wharton (41) favored the concept that *Borrelia* developed with acarinae, primarily as a parasite of these ticks, and evolved into different strains with the genetic changes that differentiated the various *Ornithodoros* species. Mammals are merely accidental hosts of borreliae according to this concept—this seems to be accepted by most writers.

Morphology

According to the majority of observers (132, 303, 363, 364, and others), borreliae are helical organisms, 3 to 25 μ long, usually 10 to 20, and 0.2 to 0.5 μ wide according to their environment and the time that has elapsed since division. Forms as short as 8 μ and as long as 40 μ have been described. They have 4 to 30 coils which are uneven, especially when the smears have been dried. Manson and Thornton (467) in Indochina and Sibilia (646) in Ethiopia reported short as well as long forms, whereas Hindle (364) described slender organisms in Central Africa. Passage through animals may result in the appearance of thicker variants (69). Aristowsky and Hoeltzer (24) observed irregular, bizarre spirals. Such forms and fragmented, conglomerating borreliae are not rare in the blood of relapsing fever patients just before the crisis. They vary in appearance (and antigenicity) during subsequent attacks in the same person (669), but variations are even more frequent when an unnatural mammalian host is inoculated with them (687). In dark field microscopy, Baltazard (47) saw a luminous contour around some strains instead of the usually uniform refraction.

Flagella were described in a so-called *B. novyi* strain maintained in the laboratory by rat passages (441). This finding was not confirmed by electron microscopy. The structure of *B. novyi* was studied by Lofgren and Soule (456), who saw a terminal filament and fragile fibers, as well as fixed and free granules in the protoplasm. Further electron microscopic studies were carried out by several other investigators (34, 35, 38, 109, 401, 402, 403, 498, 673). A foamy envelope that could be washed off with sodium deoxycholate, a cell wall formed by 2 membranes with 20 to 25 fibrils on its surface, no mitochondria, but no limiting membrane between cytoplasm and nuclear zone were seen. The cytoplasm became invaginated before cell division that took place by transverse fission. An activator membrane was also described that, according to Mölbert (498), is connected with the band of fibrils.

Pillot *et al.* (574, 575, 576) undertook a systematic study of *Treponema, Borrelia,* and *Leptospira.* All Spirochetaceae appeared to have an elastic envelope containing lipids, polyosides, and pro-

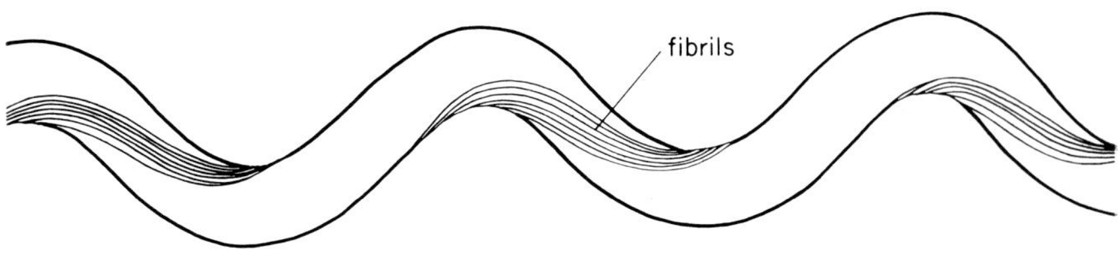

FIGURE 2. Structure of *Borrelia,* longitudinal view. Schematic drawing.

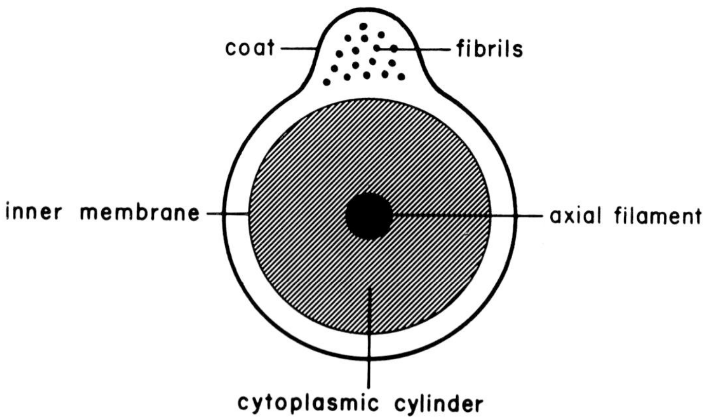

FIGURE 3. Structure of *Borrelia.* Cross section. Schematic drawing.

teins. Specific antigen is carried by the polyoside-lipid complex. The limiting cell body (parieto-cytoplasmic) membrane gives the organisms their helical shape and confines the protoplasm. It contains glucosamine peptides which confer solidity to it. The locomotory apparatus is situated between the envelope and the cytoplasmic membrane, consisting of parallel fibrils, which are coiled around the cell body. The fibrils and the cell body rotate at the same rate but in opposite directions. Intracytoplasmic mitochondria were not observed but mesosome-like structures were present. A long fibrillar nucleus without a limiting membrane was also seen. Aeschlimann *et al.* (10) studied blood forms of *B. duttonii, B. tillae, B. crocidurae,* and *B. hispanica,* as well as *B. duttonii* in *O. moubata,* with the aid of the electron microscope. An outer coat enclosing the central cytoplasmic core, with a lateral ridge running along the entire body of the organisms and harboring 15 to 22 fibrils, a cytoplasm with its own membrane and ribosomes, a central nuclear substance without membrane but running through the entire body and containing DNA were found in all examined species. *B. tillae* had an additional membrane, probably part of a mesosome. There was some difference in the degree of wrinkling of the outer membrane but no additional characteristics that would permit strain differential diagnostic characterising of the genus *Borrelia* were found. However, *Leptospira* having only one fibril, *Treponema* 3 to 7, and *Cristispira* with several hundred fibrils were encountered. Geigy (303) pointed out that the fibrils attached to granules may be similar to bacterial flagella. During cell division, each fibril has to split separately.

Electron microscopic studies put an end to the "granule" theory, which was promulgated by Leishman in 1907 (442) and Hindle in 1911 (361). It was believed that either "invisible," "filtrable," or "granular" forms represented a metacyclic development of borreliae because these organisms disappear from the blood between attacks, as well as from the gut of the vectors before they are found in the celomic fluid. Todd (685) and Leishman (442) reviewed the debate on granules; Baltazard and Habibi (58) on invisible or filtrable forms; Baltazard *et al.* (51), and Weyer (724) on metacyclic changes in general. Chorine and Crogue (169) called attention to the fact that short and small forms and presence of organisms too few to be noted may be the reason for misinterpreted morphologic intravital changes in size and numbers. Heisch *et al.* (349, 353, 355) considered granules appearing in lice to be breakdown products. Burgdorfer (129) took a firm stand against the metacyclic theory while he observed a reduction in size of *B. duttonii* during its passage in the tick. Westphal (723), using the phase microscope, saw internal segmentation of borreliae that may give rise to granule-like fractions. Felsenfeld (264) studied granules which appeared as breakdown products and involution forms rather than stages of a metacyclic process in *B. turicatae,* under the fluorescent microscope. It is not believed therefore that borreliae undergo an evolutionary life cycle in the vector or in the host.

Hindle (363, 364) described the motion of these flexible organisms that are endowed with anterioposterior polarity (243) as cork-screw like, in forward and backward waves, and laterally by bending and looping. Geigy (303) emphasized the corkscrew-like motion as permitting the penetration of the organisms through mucous membranes and even through the skin. In the body, borreliae live in extracellular and interstitial fluid but may penetrate into cells. However, they do not enter red blood cells. Under the conventional light microscope, locomotion that may be suddenly reversed, and helical rotation and twisting, are usually seen. Ackermann and Protasov (1) studied the ring-like twisting of borreliae frequently seen during the last hours of the relapse and concluded that it is a protective measure for these organisms.

Multiplication takes place by transverse fission. Unusually long forms are due to lack of separation of the daughter cells. Details are described under electron microscopic observations above.

Biochemistry

Biochemical characteristics of borreliae as determined by electron microscopic methods were described in the preceding chapter. Studies by other methods are hampered by difficulties in culturing *Borrelia,* as pointed out by Geiman (314). Nevertheless, Fenyvessy and Scheff (272) found that dextrose is utilized by glycolysis. Cell-free extracts and homogenates of *B. recurrentis* follow the Embden-Meyerhof pathway (385). Oxygen is not utilized. The so-called *B. novyi* also utilizes dextrose but accumulates excess lactic acid

(626). Scheff and Kutner (627) studied the dehydrogenase activities of *B. recurrentis*. Smith (653, 654) demonstrated in *B. recurrentis* homogenates hexokinase, P-glucoisomerase, P-fructokinase, aldolase, P-glyceraldehyde dehydrogenase, triose P-glycerate kinase, P-glyceromutase, enolase, pyruvate kinase, and DPN-dependent lactic dehydrogenase.

Both live and killed borreliae moved toward the cathode in the electric field (273).

Ginger (318) attacked the problem of classification of borreliae by biochemical means. Van Thiel (682) considered them protozoa; Lewin Cyanophyceae. Ginger chose the study of cell wall mucopeptides as a pivotal point. These yield, on hydrolysis, amino acids and sugar together with amino sugar glucosamine, galactosamine, and muramic acid. Muramic acid is present in true bacteria, Actinomycetales, Cyanophyceae, and Rickettsiae. Muramic acid was present in the *B. duttonii* strain tested by Ginger. It was also susceptible to those antibiotics that inhibit bacteria and was sensitive to lysozyme, which is a characteristic of bacteria. Moreover, there was a cell wall, and resistance to nuclear staining methods, which are not found in protozoa.

Felsenfeld *et al.* (265) studied the biochemical and physical properties of the antigenic fractions of *B. parkerii*. Two protide fractions were relapse-specific, the third common to borreliae.

It is evident that the problem of biochemical composition and metabolism of *Borrelia* requires much further study.

Immunology and Serology

Classifying *Borrelia* serologically is a very difficult task. Jancsó (383) compared the characteristics of strains collected from different relapses in the same patient, and found that cross-immunologic phenomena are not the rule. This led to recognition of the fact that borreliae undergo phase variation and develop antigenic variations during subsequent attacks by the same organism in man and animals. Beck (70) saw similar results using the protection test by inoculating animals previously infected with homologous strains collected from subsequent attacks. Several investigators (264, 303, 364, 365, 619, 630, 667 and others) reviewed this problem. Russell (618) attempted to establish "serotypes" (phases) and designated them by the use of capital letters. Experimenting with large West African rats *(Cricetomys gambianus),* she found that only serotypes A and B conferred life-long immunity. In later investigations Russell (619) found that the serotype of the variant strain recovered from a later relapse in the rat that has been inoculated with the variant will be serologically identical to the organism isolated from the patient during the attack that followed the relapse from which the *Borrelia* was originally isolated. She concluded that *Borrelia* can adapt itself repeatedly to the antibodies of the animal although the number of re-adaptations is limited.

Ashbel (28) studied 17 strains of *B. persica* in 110 guinea pigs which are strongly susceptible to this *Borrelia* strain. He found that immunologic variants occur more often in man than in animals. Serologic variants have been observed also in monkeys, and in one tick vector. The original *Borrelia* strain did not protect against infection with relapse strains in some instances. However, relapses occurred with and without the development of variants.

Schuhardt and Wilkerson (632) infected rats with single organisms of *B. turicatae* and found that serologically different variants emerged. The immobilizines and lysins that developed against them were different, however. In man, Sterling-Okunewski (669) noted that serologic variants appeared in consecutive attacks regardless of the number of circulating borreliae. Ackermann and Protasov (1) considered it possible that the immunity conferred by the first attack affords only relative protection. Schuhardt (630, 631) defined the relapse phenomenon as the result of the inherent capacity of borreliae to undergo one or more antigenic variations. Cunningham (211) stated that there is a tendency to revert to a previous variant phase during subsequent relapses and that the dominant phase may be stable or not in various strains.

Cunningham *et al.* (213) experimented on squirrels *(Sciurus palmaris)* and monkeys. They described 9 phases and labeled them according to their sequence in consecutive attacks, from A to I. Phase A from the first attack, B from the first relapse, and D and E from the second relapse were complementary to each other. Phase C from a second attack in a mixed infection, and D and E from the second relapse were related to B; phase G from a second attack was related to phase A. Phase F was rare, whereas, H and I developed in prolonged relapses, when phase B was at a low ebb. In man, mostly A and B were observed, with C, F, and G occurring less often, and with a tendency to revert to A or B. This study demonstrated the intricacies of the serologic structure as well as the coexistence of several variants. The practical application of the finding of more stable phases was tested by Cunningham and Fraser (212) on the Northwest Frontier of India. Most sera in that area did not react with phase B of the louse-borne *Borrelia.* Type C gave positive reactions.

Tick-borne borreliae appear to undergo more variations than louse-borne species. Coffey and Eveland (185) described 4 subsequently developing serotypes of *B. hermsii.* They designated them O - A - B - C. A tendency to revert to phase O was noted. Variants were also found in ticks by Cunningham and Fraser (212). Some investigators do not agree with these authors (28). Neither the antigenic schedules of Cunningham nor the six phases of *B. recurrentis* of Meleney (490) who studied *B. recurrentis* in splenectomized squirrels *(Sciurotamias davidianus)* and chipmunks *(Eutamias asiaticus)* attained popularity, even though the latter emphasized only phases A and B which he found reversible. Considering that Toyoda (688) observed phase variations also depending on the treatment of the patients, the great number of strains, substrains, and mutants, all of them producing a number of different variants under varying conditions delineated by their own microclimate, one has to agree that extreme caution is necessary in making generalizations from limited studies. Unfortunately, type collections of borreliae do not exist to the knowledge of this author. This hinders even further comparative and comprehensive studies of this aspect of borreliosis.

Serologic and other studies of borreliae are further impeded by the occurrence of partly related, partly dissimilar strains in the same locality or in nearby localities. Some instances have been mentioned previously. Dubois (247) observed such strains within the radius of 80 kilometers in the Congoes. Geigy and Burgdorfer (303, 307) had a similar experience with *B. duttonii* strain labeled B. Infection protected mice against strains C and D but not *vice versa.* They called this a one-sided immunity. Addamiano and Babudieri (2) observed the same phenomenon with two strains designated Irbid and Husu, respectively, in Jordan, and coined the term "asymmetric immunity." Cross-protection between different species, at least to a moderate degree, was described among members of the crocidurae subgroup (188), in bush-babies and not regularly in primates between *B. recurrentis* and *B. duttonii* (296), and not between *B. recurrentis, B. duttonii,* and the North American tick-borne species (193, 194). Thus cross-protection is not always the rule. Reciprocal immunity may or may not be present. This restricts the value of neutralization and cross-protection tests in animals.

Serologic methods feasible for routine laboratory work were reviewed by Schuhardt (630) and Wilson and Miles (735). They disagree on the value of the agglutination test. It appears that a feasible agglutination or precipitation test has yet to be developed because technical difficulties, principally the limited number of organisms available, the complexity of the test in Treponemataceae (363, 364), cross-reactions with *Treponema* (12, 623), and auto-agglutination thwart efforts to demonstrate agglutinins with ease and certainty.

Brussin (125) studied the adhesin phenomenon. It was found feasible for pratical use when only few borreliae are present in the blood (630). Adhesins appear later during the disease (364). Adler and Ashbel (3) described a factor causing adhesion of borreliae to leukocytes and, if the protoplasm of these cells is destroyed, also to white blood cell nuclei. Adhesin is independent from lysin in *B. turicatae* and *B. parkerii* (265). Mooser (500) observed that *B. duttonii* show mutual adhesion, and display this phenomenon not only with leukocytes but also with red blood cells, and on the bare surface of slides and coverslips. He was able to prevent adhesin activity by homologous but not by heterologous serum.

Borrelia enters leukocytes even in the absence of phagocytic activity, by pinocytosis. While Adler and Ashbel (3) did not observe phagocytosis, Belezki and Umanskaia (72) recorded some such activity by elements of the reticuloendothelial system (RES), including monocytes and histiocytes. In the central nervous system, glia cells and Hortega cells acted as phagocytes. Similar relationships exist in mice, after RES blockade and splenectomy (126).

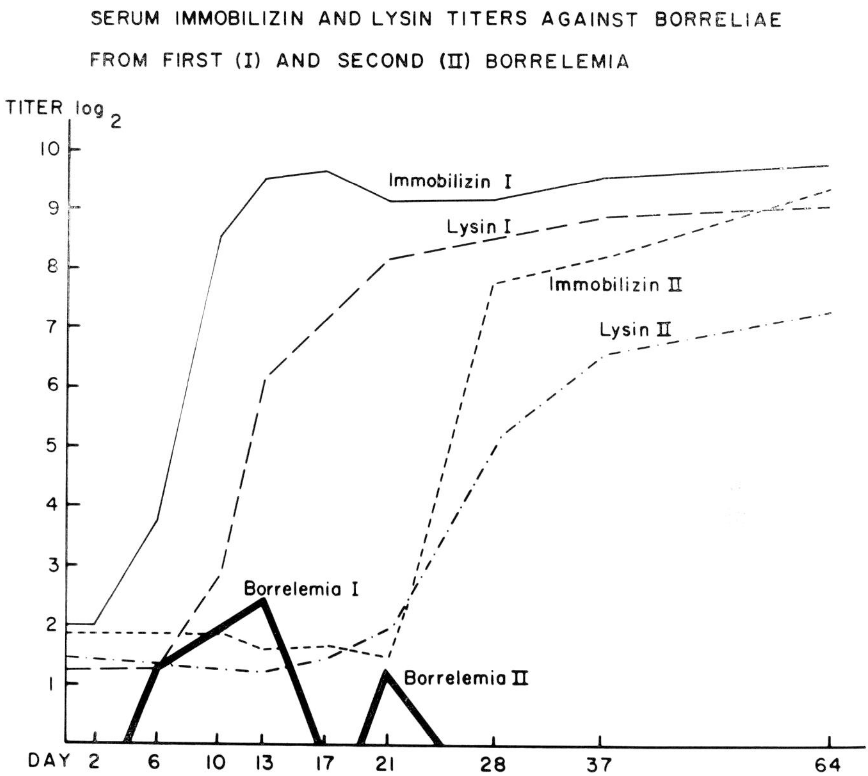

FIGURE 4. Serologic data, patas monkey *(Erythrocebus patas)* infected with *Borrelia parkerii.*

Immobilizines were said to be of small molecular size (449) and are related to β and γ globulins (136). They were observed also in the heavy (19S) IgM (268). Immobilizines can be found in the serum long after the infection has subsided (268, 449, 450) and may be directed against a specific phase of the causative agent (598). These antibodies are present also during the latent phases of the disease. They are strain specific (697). Levaditi *et al.* (450) expressed the opinion that antibodies such as immobilizines may induce phase variation in borreliae.

The borreliolytic activity of the serum of infected man and animals appears to be identical to antiborrelial cytolysin and borreliocidin (262). It was considered inconstant in guinea pigs infected with *B. hispanica* but in man it persisted for nearly a year

(572). Toyoda (688) had the same experience. Ranque *et al.* (597, 599) found it highly specific, whereas complement fixation test, fluorescent microscopy, and skin tests showed cross-reactions. The cardiolipid hapten and group proteins are, however, common to related organisms.

Toyoda (688) and Wolstenholme and Gear (737) described complement fixing antibodies in relapsing fever which will be further discussed in the chapter on Laboratory Diagnosis.

Immunity to borreliae has been termed a premunition-like phenomenon by Geigy and Burgdorfer (307). The studies of Chamsa (153) led him to the conclusion that this premunition is strain specific.

Loewy (455) correlated the periodic changes of body temperature during relapses ending with crisis, and the lesions often observed in the nervous system in the course of the disease, principally when treatment has been started late. Therefore, he concluded that anaphylactic phenomena play a role in relapsing fever.

Little has been said about natural antibodies in borreliosis. Weichbrodt (719) questioned whether they may not be present in the cerebrospinal fluid. Such antibodies, or the lack of some physiologic capabilities of certain *Borrelia* strains, could explain why not all borreliae invade the central nervous system.

Staining

Borreliae have an affinity for acid dyes, whereas many other bacteria prefer basic dyes (720). Nevertheless, borreliae can be stained with practically any aniline dye (132). Azur-eosine and related stains of Leishman, Giemsa, May-Grünwald, Romanowski, Wright, and their combinations are favored for staining blood films from patients and animals.

Du (246) described a simple and effective method feasible also for the staining of thick blood smears. The slides are dehemoglobinized with 6% acetic acid in 95% ethanol, rinsed, and then stained with carbolfuchsin for 1 minute.

Pampana (561) stained thick drops with a 2% methylene blue B extra solution in distilled water, to which 4 ml formol and 10 ml glacial acetic acid were added after filtration. Methylene blue was used also by Simons (648) who mixed 1 ml saturated methylene blue solution in physiologic saline with 2 ml 10% sodium taurocholate in saline, added 2 to 4 loopfuls of this mixture to an equal volume of blood, then made smears with it on microscope slides. This method can be used also for the examination of citrated blood which first has to be centrifuged and then the sediment can be examined.

As most workers do who use routine blood stains, Coles (196) also recommended prolonged staining but employed orange tannin for differentiation after the coloration. Vago (696) and Young (743) recommended mercurochrome. The latter employed concentrated aqueous mercurochrome for 3 minutes, followed by concentrated aqueous methyl violet. Our group (264) applied 1% crystal violet for a few seconds after staining according to Wright. Other combinations, such as the use of saturated alcoholic or aqueous solutions of a basic dye followed by an acid dye in 30% alcohol (gentian violet and acid green, or brilliant green and acid fuchsin) were recommended by Weiss (720). Levine (451) used careful fixation of airdried smears, first with acid-free chloroform, then with acid-free absolute ethanol. Fuchsin was recommended for staining.

Fluorescent antibody studies of borreliae were made by Coffey and Eveland (184) who found them superior to the immobilizine and lysin tests. Maestrone (463) used the fluorescent antibody method for leptospiral and viral antigens in formol-fixed tissues that is applicable also to borreliae. The tissues are re-fixed with acetone for 5 minutes, dried at 37° C, exposed to ammonia vapors for 2 days at 37° C, or acted upon with 1% ammonia for 3 to 5 minutes. Sodium bisulfite, 25% for 5 minutes, may be substituted. The slides are washed with 3% Tween 80 containing saline buffer pH 7.2, blotted dry, reacted with rabbit anti-*Borrelia* serum or globulin, then, after washing with buffered saline, sandwiched with a fluorescein isocyanate or rhodamine labeled anti-rabbit serum, and mounted in glycerol. A slight shrinkage is usually apparent.

Silver impregnation methods are used for the visualization of borreliae in tissues. That of Krajian gives excellent results and will be described in the Appendix in detail.

The methods of choice will be discussed in the chapter Laboratory Diagnosis.

Culture Methods

In Vitro

Noguchi (544, 545) succeeded in growing *B. recurrentis* and *B. duttonii* in a rabbit kidney-ascitic fluid medium, under liquid paraffin seal. Maximal growth was observed in 7 to 9 days. First short, then longitudinally dividing forms were seen. Noguchi succeeded in passing the Koch strain 29 times over a period of about 6 months in this medium but others (262, 513) were not successful in attempts to culture borreliae from the blood and organs of patients using this medium. Others (658) had better results with laboratory strains. Kligler and Robertson (414) pointed out that the medium should be slightly alkaline. These authors used ascitic fluid, horse or rabbit serum, 1% peptone broth, or egg albumin solution. Moroder (504) employed a mixture of inactivated rabbit or horse serum with 2 to 5 parts of physiologic saline, and covered the cultures with liquid paraffin. Granules still present in old cultures were infective for mice. Li (452) dispersed the yolk of one egg in 400 ml physiologic saline and added egg white. After coagulation, liquid paraffin was layered over the slants. One or 2 drops of citrated blood were put into the supernate when transfers were made. Chorine and Crogue (169) also used blood. Their medium contained peptone water, fresh rabbit serum, Tyrode's solution (which could be omitted), and laked or defibrinated human blood. It took 7 to 8 passages to establish the slowly growing strains. Others (44) were not successful with the medium of Chorine and Crogue.

Wolman and Wolman (736) prepared their medium by adding 10 ml human ascitic fluid to 1 ml coagulated egg albumen. An equal volume of buffer pH 7.8 and 2 volumes of 1% dextrose were added. After covering with liquid paraffin, the mixture was held at 56° C for 1 hour each on 3 consecutive days. *B. recurrentis* lived and multiplied in this medium for 8 months but lost its virulence after a year. Krylova (426) had good results with a modified Wolman procedure.

It should be noted that most authors who succeeded in growing borreliae *in vitro* did so at 28° to 30° C, or at even lower temperatures.

There is little hope that any of these methods could be used successfully in routine diagnostic laboratories. Further investigations may lead to the development of more feasible methods.

In Developing Chick Embryos

Chabaud (150) inoculated *B. recurrentis* and *B. duttonii*-containing defibrinated and centrifuged blood on the chorioallantoic membrane (CAM). The organisms multiplied after 3 to 5 days but the embryos died on the 6th to 7th day. The incubation period was reduced after repeated passages. Experiments with defibrinated blood were more successful than with citrated blood. Oag (549) reported in the same year that *B. duttonii* does not cause the death of developing chick embryos. The motility but not the virulence of the organisms increased after serial transfers. Later (550) Oag found that when chick embryos were inoculated 2 to 3 days before hatching, the borreliae were detectable in the blood of the chickens for about 5 days. Blood or serum from mice and fowl and of the chick embryo was borreliocidal *in vitro* but not *in vivo*. Oag could not offer an explanation for this phenomenon.

Other authors (91, 158, 334) were satisfied with the feasibility of chick embryos to support the propagation of borreliae, principally when inoculating 7 to 12 day old fertilized eggs. More than 35 passages were possible in 4 months (334). The use of fertilized chick embryos, inoculating them either just under the CAM or into the yolk sac, has become an important diagnostic aid because relatively few animals are susceptible to *B. recurrentis*. Chen (158) observed growth on the 5th day but the borreliae also died when the eggs expired. Rodhain and van den Bergh (609) stated that borreliae that attack adult fowl do not grow in developing chick embryos but that *B. duttonii* gave good results in 10 day old embryos. Several investigators (40, 44, 76) were satisfied with this method but found the transferability somewhat irregular.

Tissue Cultures

Manteufel and Dressler (468) prepared tissue cultures from allantoic membranes and found that *B. hispanica* multiplied on them. Our group has been studying the adaptability of *B. turicatae* to several cell lines but without much success.

Maintenance at Low Temperature

Sparrow (665) called attention to the numerous factors that influence the survival and the virulence of borreliae, particularly of *B. recurrentis*. Geigy and Sarasin (310) discussed the control exerted by the environment over *B. duttonii*. While Hindle (364) stated that borreliae survived only about one day in sealed slide preparations, they could be kept alive in citrated blood for 3 months at 0° to 2° C but were killed in 30 minutes at 50°. Ackermann and Protasov (1) found that borreliae retained their virulence in the refrigerator for more than 100 days but Hindle (364) observed a gradual diminution in the number that remained virulent. Beck (69) found that North American borreliae died in frozen animal tissues after a few days but survived in sheep blood for more than 6 months. Bourgain (105, 106) kept *B. persica* alive at 4° C for 19 days, at 11° to 15° C for 7, and at at 37° C for 4 days. They died in isolated mammalian organs in the refrigerator in 7 days but in cadavers at room temperatures in 4 days. Temperatures between —15° and —20° C killed them in 2 days, whereas others (726) kept borreliae alive at —72° C for several years. Kemp *et al.* (405) found, however, that *B. turicatae* is killed by sodium citrate used to keep the blood from coagulating, and by freezing. Beck (69) also preferred refrigeration to freezing. Hanson and Cannefax (336) recommended lyophilization as a means of preserving borreliae. Lofgren and Soule (456) destroyed borreliae by repeated freezing and thawing.

Borrel and Marchoux (103) found that borreliae multiply best in ticks at 35° C. Leishman (442) also stated that borreliae degenerate in ticks more rapidly at lower temperatures. These observations are of importance for the understanding of the seasonal fluctuations of tick-borne relapsing fever.

These and similar findings, coupled with the tediousness of the attempts at culturing borreliae in test tubes or in developing chick embryos, led to experiments directed at maintaining them in their vectors and hosts.

Maintenance in Vectors and Host Organs

The longevity of some ticks carrying borreliae is remarkable.

Pavlovskii and Skrynnik (569) kept *O. tholozani* alive for 16 years at 15° to 18° C. They had to be fed only once a year. Larval stages could starve 15 months; nymphs 2 to 11 years; and adults 10 years. Pavlovskii and Skrynnik (568) also observed that *O. tholozani* could starve 7½ years and remain alive, transmit *B. persica* after 12 years, and live for 25 years. Mooser (501) found *O. moubata* alive and carrying its *Borrelia* for 2 years. Brumpt (120) stated that borreliae can be preserved in their vectors at 5° to 7° C for several weeks, without loss of virulence.

It has become common laboratory practice to keep ticks infected with borreliae in a sandbox, or in test tubes with a strip of filter paper running along the center of the tubes. The ticks are fed on young, preferably newborn mice. If dead animals are offered for food (the *Ornithodoros* ticks live only on blood), the cadaver may be put into the sandbox ("tickorium"). Not all individuals in the colony will be infected or transmit borreliae to their progeny. The maintenance of proper humidity may cause difficulties. Nevertheless, the long survival of borreliae in their vectors is an excellent means of keeping them alive, handy, and ready in the laboratory.

Another method of maintaining borreliae in the laboratory is preservation in the brains of infected rodents. Ashbel (28) was able to preserve *B. persica* in guinea pig brains for 380 days. Toda and Hiroki (683) failed in their attempts at preserving the Manchurian strain of *B. recurrentis* in mouse brain. Delpy and Rafyi (235) stated that guinea pigs are not susceptible to louse-borne borreliae but only to the tick-borne strains. They were able to maintain *B. persica* in mammalian brain for 8 to 73 days. Sergent (640) transmitted *B. hispanica* and found it in a guinea pig brain 3 years after it had disappeared from the blood. Mathis and Durieux (479) made passages of *B. duttonii* in animals every 3 to 4 weeks. Fatal infection did not ensue, but inoculation of infective blood did kill the recipient mice. Pirot and Bourgain (579) called attention to individual variations in the susceptibility of guinea pigs. Some of the guinea pigs lived more than 7 months, in others the cerebral infection disappeared in 45 days. Sergent and Poncet (643) experimented with *B. hispanica* in rats for which it was less frequently fatal than for guinea pigs. The route of inoculation greatly influenced the outcome of the research, the subcutaneous inoculation causing appearance of fewer borreliae in the blood than intraperitoneal administration of the organisms.

Pampana (561) sacrificed guinea pigs 6 months after infection, using chloroform, washed the brains with saline, emulsified them, and then injected the emulsion into fresh animals. The incubation period was 6 to 12 days.

Weyer (725) studied different methods of preserving *B. duttonii, B. turicatae,* and *B. crocidurae.* They remained alive when quick frozen at −76° C. *B. recurrentis* in lice, and tick-borne in *Ornithodoros,* remained alive in the deep freeze for years. Even more effective was the propagation of *B. recurrentis* by inoculation into the hemolymph of lice. When borreliae were numerous, they could be frozen in rat blood. Weyer's method can be recommended provided the arthropods are not thawed and refrozen.

BORRELIAE AND THEIR VECTORS

It will be seen on subsequent pages that it is difficult, perhaps even impossible, to speak about species of *Borrelia.* All of these so-called species may well be the variants of one single organism adapted to different environments programmed by vectors, hosts, and their mutual relationship. However, following the present custom of classifying borreliae according to their vectors (which is of considerable epidemiologic interest), the vectors will be discussed together with the "strains" they usually carry, or are said to harbor. Experiments with cross-infections of vectors will be listed, as well as strains that have been described but either were lost or were found to be mere variants of established *Borrelia* types. It is necessary to present separate discussions of the louse with *B. recurrentis* and ticks with their borreliae for reasons which are evident.

The Human Louse and Borrelia Recurrentis

As mentioned before, Mackie was the first to incriminate the human body louse as the vector of epidemic relapsing fever. Nicolle and his co-workers (531, 532, 537, 538) worked out many details of the louse-*Borrelia* relationship. Nicolle and Anderson (521) believed that the contemporary strains of *B. recurrentis* were derived from tick-borne strains. Adler and Ashbel (4) agreed with this concept.

Lice

General accounts of the life cycle of the louse and of the mode of transmission of borreliae by this insect have been given by

TABLE 2
SIZE OF SOME ARTHROPODS CARRYING BORRELIAE AND THEIR NICKNAMES+

Scientific Name	*Male**	*Female*	*Nickname*
Pediculus humanus corporis	2.5-3.3 x 0.8-1.1	3.2-3.6 x 1.1-1.4	
Pediculus humanus capitis	1.6-2.1 x 0.6-0.8	2.4-2.8 x 0.9-1.1	
Ornithodoros moubata	4.2-5.8 x 3.7-4.2	7.8-12.8 x 6.9-10.2	Ochiopo, Tampan, Garrapato (Angola) Kufu, Bu (Zambezia) Kibu, Bibo (Uganda) Papasi (Zanzibar) Kimputu (Congoes) Curdud (Somaliland)
Ornithodoros erraticus	2.8-4.2 x 1.8-2.5	4.2-6.8 x 2.4-4.1	
Ornithodoros tholozani	3.5-6.2 x 2.8-5.2	7.6-9.1 6.8-7.4	
Ornithodoros rudis	3.3-4.2 x 2.4-3.3	4.8-6.4 x 2.8-4.2	Cuescas, Mordijini (Venezuela) Talajas (Colombia)
Ornithodoros talaje	4.8-6.2 x 3.4-5.2	5.3-7.4 x 4.7-6.2	
Ornithodoros turicata	2.7-4.4 x 2.3-2.9	4.6-6.9 x 3.3-4.3	Pajaroello (Mexico)
Argas persicus	4.0-5.5 x 2.6-3.3	5.0-10.1 2.4-7.5	

* In mm, length x width.

Size often depends on time since last feeding.

+ Nicknames according to Brumpt, E.: *Précis de Parasitologie,* 6th ed. Mason & Cie., Paris, 1963.

numerous authors. Nicolle *et al.* (534) found that the organisms are not transmitted to the progeny of lice. Chapcheff (155) and Chiao (163) emphasized that only *Pediculus humanus corporis (vestimenti)* and *Pediculus humanus capitis,* i.e., the clothes or body louse, and the head louse, respectively, but not the pubic or crab louse, *Phthirus pubis,* transfer relapsing fever organisms.This was confirmed by data in the monograph on lice by Buxton (135) and in the textbook of Horsfall (374). Thus we are concerned only with the human body louse and the closely related head louse.

The genus *Pediculus* is a member of the family Pediculidae that belongs to the order Anoplura (Siphunculata) or sucking lice. The body louse, *P. h. corporis* is also called *P. humanus humanus.* The head louse is about 2.5 mm long and slightly smaller than the body louse but they can interbreed. Lice are strictly host-specific. Geigy (303) stated that head lice must have preceded body lice and adjusted themselves to man before he started to wear clothing. Lice cling to hair. The body louse does not invade the head hair and beard but *P. h. capitis* may migrate to the body. *P. h. corporis* lives also in the folds of clothing, principally in the underwear. The fertilized female lays about 300 eggs which adhere to hair or cloth-

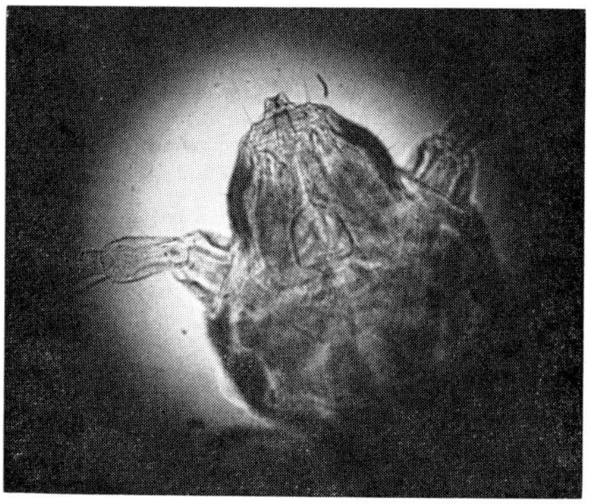

FIGURE 5. Head of louse, *Pediculus humanus.*

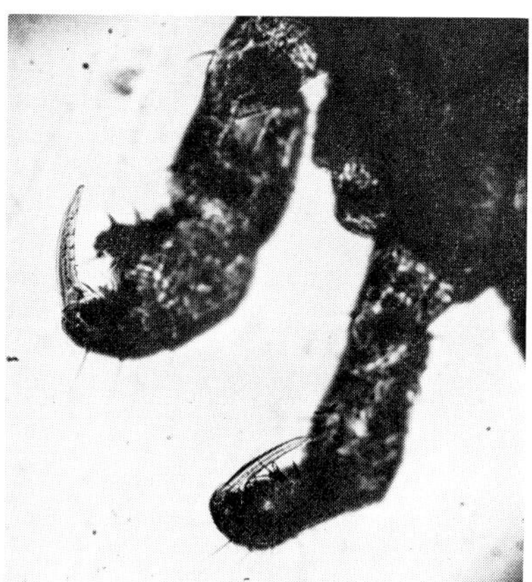

FIGURE 6. Claws of human louse, *Pediculus humanus.*

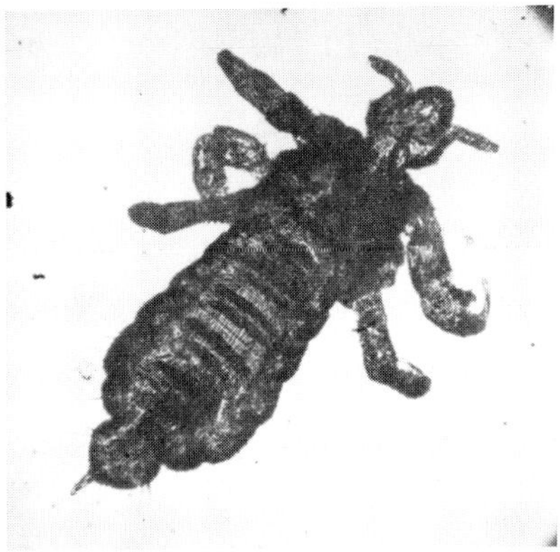

FIGURE 7. Male louse, *Pediculus humanus (corporis).*

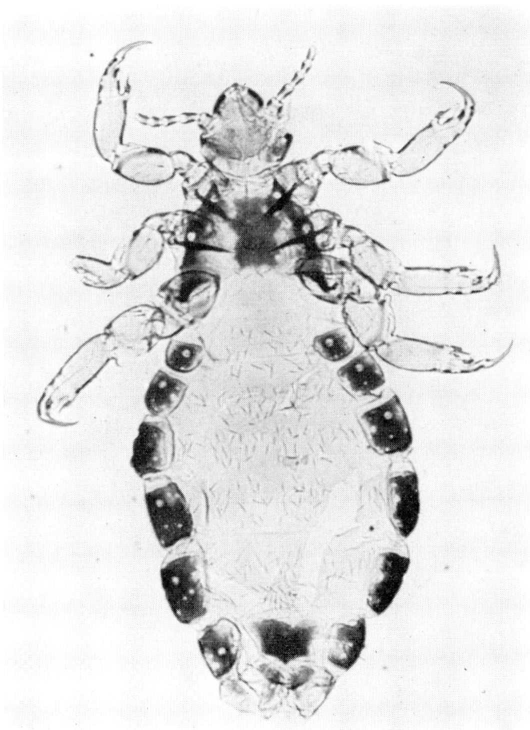

FIGURE 8. Human louse, *Pediculus humanus (corporis),* female. Slide preparation.

ing and hatch at 28° to 32° C in 8 to 9 days. Three larval stages develop within 9 to 10 days. The larvae and nymphs descend to the skin and feed. One adult louse takes up about 1 mg blood at one meal but it is possible that smaller amounts are consumed and then the lice feed more often. Feeding is rapid and followed by a quick evacuation of feces. If the louse has a meal on a patient with *B. recurrentis* in his blood, the organisms reach the stomach of the louse but many are destroyed. Heisch *et al.* (355) found that the density of the borreliae in the blood consumed by the louse must be at least one or two per oil immersion field to make the meal infective.

The borreliae pass from the gut into the hemocele (celomic cavity) where they multiply. In the louse, organs like the salivary glands, the ovaries, or the Malpighian bodies are not invaded. This precludes hereditary transmission. Only about 12% of the lice fed on relapsing fever patients became infected in the experiments of Nicolle *et al.* (534). In one instance 4,407 lice were fed on a patient, and none acquired borreliae. On the other hand, Riding and MacDowell (603) found that one-half of the lice that were collected from persons who were ill with relapsing fever for 1 to 10 days were infected with borreliae. The organisms become visible in the celomic fluid (hemolymph) about 5 to 8 days after the blood meal. The borreliae remain in the louse until its death. Since borreliae are not present in the gut and salivary glands, they cannot be transmitted by the bite of the louse. Neither can they be propagated by fecal material. Borreliae may escape from the celomic cavity only when the louse is crushed (179).

Heisch and Harvey (353) described several basic data on the relationship of lice and borreliae. They showed that the hemocytes of the louse may act as phagocytes and destroy some borreliae. These authors found borreliae also in the neural ganglion and nucleus but never in the salivary gland of the louse. The penetration of the borreliae into the hemocele took place from the anterior part of the midgut.

After a blood meal containing borreliae, the organisms disappear from the midgut of the louse within a few hours, to reappear in the hemocele after 5 to 8 days. This has been called the "negative phase." It has given rise to speculations about a filtrable phase of borreliae. The appearance of granules, short and cork-screw-like forms of borreliae, in the beginning of their sojourn in the celomic cavity has stimulated speculation and research also about metacyclic forms (54, 63, 296, 348, 353, 355). These investigations showed that a metacyclic development does not exist in the louse. The organisms become slender and small when penetrating the midgut but they can be found by diligent search. The "granula" theory is difficult to prove or disprove except with the aid of fluorescent microscopy, as our group did (264), because "granules" occur naturally in the celomic cavity of lice.

The number of surviving borreliae is determined by the temperature and the hitherto not fully explored qualitative and quantitative changes of the gut juices of the louse. Wolman and Wolman (736) found, for instance, that lice kept at 37° C were unable to infect man 1 to 18 days after a meal on a patient with relapsing fever.

The borreliae are tightly enclosed by the limiting membranes of the celomic cavity. Lice are delicate, however, and easily damaged. Their limbs and antennae are easily broken off. This permits the celomic fluid to flow out and to infect the site of the bite. This usually happens when a bitten person scratches himself. Scratching will also rub the borreliae into the skin (179, 537, 538). Small children develop relapsing fever less often than adults. This may be because they seldom crush lice. In Europe, lice are crushed between thumbnails. In China and South America, lice are often popped between the teeth. A few authors (177) believe that putting lice into the mouth does not convey the infection but it has been shown (59, 365) that borreliae may enter the human body through uninjured mucosae, including that of the gastrointestinal tract. The last practice may therefore lead to an increased number of relapsing fever infections.

After acquiring *B. recurrentis,* the louse remains infectious for its entire life, which is about 3 weeks, sometimes longer (63, 134, 453).

Experiments with louse-borne relapsing fever are hampered by the unwillingness of the human louse to bite other animals, except monkeys (59, 95, 532). It has also been reported that it is possible to feed human lice on newborn rabbits and other newborn rodents (208, 209, 219).

Human lice have a narrow temperature tolerance and die when

it becomes too hot (207). This has epidemiologic significance, which will be discussed later.

"Strains" of B. recurrentis

Coleman (194) emphasized strain specificity but pointed out pitfalls encountered in cross-protection tests. Chen *et al.* (160) used hamsters and monkeys to ascertain whether the Chinese and the American strains are identical with the aid of such tests.

Without the benefit of strain comparison, a *Borrelia* was isolated from a patient with relapsing fever at Bellevue Hospital in New York in 1907. This strain has been kept in numerous laboratories and used in animal and biochemical experiments. It is not known whether it was louse- or tick-borne. After literally thousands of rodent passages, this strain is widely used as a model for laboratory experimentation with borreliae under the designation *B. novyi*. It is not certain whether conclusions reached from experiments with this "strain" are valid for other borreliae.

It was clear to Noguchi as early as 1912 that *B. kochi* Novy 1907 was closely related to *B. rossi* Nuttal 1908, and that both organisms, as well as *B. carteri* Mackie 1907 and *B. berbera* Sergent and Foley 1910, were local strains of *B. recurrentis*. The author (O.F.) has been unable to find any laboratory that is still carrying either of these four strains. The description of *B. aegyptica* is not clear enough to warrant its acceptance as a "species."

It is possible that some or all of these strains were tick-borne rather than louse-borne. Nicolle and Anderson (520), working in Tunisia, believed that louse-borne borreliae can be transferred to ticks.

Baltazard and his co-workers (52) carried out extensive experiments by feeding lice and ticks on newborn rabbits artificially infected with borreliae. They found that lice could acquire infestation with *B. microti, B. turicatae,* and *B. hermsii* by sucking blood of infant rabbits infected with these tick-borne strains. Numerous metacyclic forms appeared in lice infested by this method. Heisch and Garnham (349) fed batches of lice from a relapsing fever-free area (Nairobi) on monkeys infected with a *B. duttonii* strain. The so-called negative phase (absence of visible forms in the insect) was shorter than in ticks; and the organisms appeared in metacyclic, cork-screw forms. This observation is important in the study of transmission of borreliosis because Heisch and Garnham found persons infested with lice living in huts in which *O. moubata*, the carrier of *B. duttonii*, was a common inhabitant. Heisch (341) believed, therefore, that the human louse can transmit *B. duttonii* under natural conditions. Heisch (346, 347) also noted a definite multiplication of *B. duttonii* in the celomic cavity of lice 6 to 8 days after ingestion. The borreliae had a tendency to concentrate around the fat body in the head of the louse. Granular forms of the *Borrelia* also appeared. This may be a phenomenon related to life in an unusual vector, and perhaps it may also be a phenomenon of adaptation. Mooser and Weyer (502) could retransmit the borreliae to *O. moubata*. *B. duttonii* did not seem to be adversely affected during 21 louse passages. Boiron (97) succeeded in transmitting *B. crocidurae, B. duttonii,* and *B. hispanica* to lice from infected mice. Weyer and Mooser (726) used rectal or intracelomic inoculation of lice, with *B. duttonii, B. turicatae,* and a crocidurae-group strain. Sparrow (660) confirmed that *B. hispanica* can be adapted to the louse, and that small rodents may become reservoirs of louse-borne tick fever. Garnham (295) believed that lice may harbor *B. hispanica* and that a man-louse-man cycle is possible, thereby forming a reservoir without passage through *O. erraticus,* the tick-vector of *B. hispanica,* and also bypassing rodents that are frequent hosts of this strain. Baltazard *et al.* (54) experimented with *B. crocidurae* and an antigenically distinct *B. microti* strain. Lice were fed on patients, tritiated, and injected into human beings and animals. Of 62 individuals and rodents, 14 became infected. Talice (675), however, did not observe infestation of lice with *B. hispanica* when fed on infected man, mice, rats, and monkeys. Favorova *et al.* (261) fed 4,658 lice on patients with tick-borne relapsing fever. The borreliae penetrated into the hemolymph in 1.25% of the lice but multiplied only in one. This group of investigators did not believe, therefore, that tick-borne borreliae can be transmitted to lice.

There appears, however, to be satisfactory evidence that tick-borne borreliae can be transmitted to lice. The antigenic stability of borreliae in insects is much greater than in animals. Probably repeated transmission cycles are required to establish variants and mutants with genetically modified characteristics that are relevant for such an adaptation . Baltazard (46) expressed this thought in considering *B. recurrentis* a transient, inconstant form of *Borrelia* that has been modified by passages in rodents and ticks. We would add to this as a governing factor the man-louse biotope.

It should be mentioned that the monkey louse *(Pediculus longiceps)* is an excellent host of *B. duttonii* (342). In view of other extensive research on *O. moubata (vide infra),* it would be perhaps somewhat rash to conclude that monkeys or *P. longiceps* play an important role in the preservation of *B. duttonii.*

Tick-borne Relapsing Fever

General Tick-Borrelia Relationships

Geigy (303) pointed out that ticks are arthropods but not insects. Ticks carrying the agent of human relapsing fever are classified in the phyllum Arthropoda, class Arachnoidea (Arachnida), order Acarina, suborder Ixodides. The order Acarina includes also spiders and scorpions. Ticks are wingless; their body lacks segmentation into head, thorax, and abdomen; and a capitulum with mouth parts and palpae is on their ventral side. They have four pairs of legs (larvae only three pairs) which are articulated and equipped with terminal claws. They have many characteristics, however, of true insects, as the Malpighian (excretory) tubules, a tracheal breathing system, and a chitinous matrix of the hypodermis.

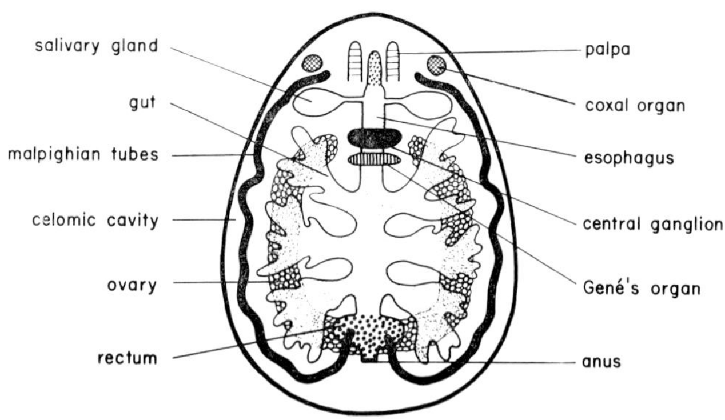

FIGURE 9. Schematic section through an *Ornithodoros.*

The suborder Ixodides consists of two main families: Ixodidae or hard ticks with 8 genera and about 400 species, and Argasidae or soft ticks, with 4 genera and about 120 species (543). Argasidae have a softer and more elastic surface than Ixodidae. They have usually only one or two principal hosts, whereas Ixodidae are willing to feed on several different animal species. Argasidae attach themselves to the host for the blood meal for only a short time and take up less blood at one feeding but their body expands considerably during the feeding. Then the females, if fertilized, lay 100 or more eggs. The number of eggs is limited (some other ticks lay them by the thousands) and the female does not die after oviposition. This fertilization and egg laying is repeated several times during life. The genus *Ornithodoros* of the family Argasidae has no scutum; the margin of the body is thick, rounded, without definite sutural line (as Argas); and the hypostome has well-developed teeth. The integument is mammillated (371, 543). *Ornithodoros* (formerly spelled *Ornithodorus*) ticks can survive for a long time without food and at a low humidity. A thin layer of wax-like substance in the epicuticle and the capability of absorbing moisture by closing the spiracles allows *Ornithodoros* to remain alive under unfavorable conditions. About 15 species of this tick have been proved to carry borreliae.

Ornithodoros feed exclusively on blood. They may ingest amounts equivalent to 2 to 6 times their own weight (438). Saliva reaches the capillaries in the skin of the bitten animal. Towards the end of the feeding the contents of the gut are evacuated through the mouth. There is no rectal outlet, only a urinary pore with a rectal bladder and two Malpighian tubes. The urinary pore is often called a rectal pore but feces are not discharged through it. Water is excreted through the coxal glands. The pressure of the engorged gut seems to aid in this process. There may be copious coxal fluid excretion (as in *O. moubata*) or only a drop which may not appear at all while the tick is in contact with its host during feeding. Normally, nymphs feed more often than adult ticks. After feeding, *Ornithodoros* leave their host.

Sautet (624) summarized the natural animal hosts of *Ornithodoros*. His studies and those of Mooser (501) and others show that *O. moubata* and the human body louse are primarily anthropophilic, whereas other ticks are parasitic principally on other animals, mainly rodents and insectivores.

There are numerous animals on which certain species of *Ornithodoros* feed. The feeding usually takes 10 to 30 minutes, seldom 1 hour or longer, according to the species of tick. The bite of some species is painful, whereas others produce analgesia. *Borrelia*-transmitting ticks usually do not have a painful bite, and feed for a relatively short time, which affords them some safety from being scratched or shaken off by the host. Baltazard *et al.* (56), discussing host-vector relationship of ticks, stated that young animals are better hosts because they are unable to rid themselves of the tick with ease. Considering the greater susceptibility and higher mortality rate of young rodents when infected with borreliae, and the willingness of *Ornithodoros* to feed also on young dead animals, the tick-rodent relationship in a given ecosystem results in the survival of the tick but in a diminishing number of their young hosts. The time of the emergence of hungry nymphs often also coincides with that of new wild rodent litters, which further contributes to the effective survival of *Ornithodoros*.

As in the louse, the borreliae penetrate into the celomic cavity of the tick. First small, thick, and cork-screw-like forms are seen, as well as thin, elongated borreliae. They have a predilection for the central ganglion, the two coxal and salivary glands, and the genitals including the gonads. This results in transovarian transmission which does not take place, however, in all instances. Borreliae pass with the eggs but not all larvae become infested (7). Details were studied by Aeschlimann (8) and Wagner-Jevseenko (708). The borreliae appear to penetrate the follicular layer around the ovules, pass through the surface of the eggs, and reach the yolk through the protoplasmic cortex. The number of infested eggs varies according to the species: up to 100% *O. turicatae,* 80% *O. moubata,* but less than 2% *O. hermsi* eggs will become infested (222, 303). Borreliae multiply during larval development and reach the salivary glands, so that first-instar (F_1) nymphs are already infested.

The organotropism is probably of chemical nature. Bruen and Blatter (104) believed that it might be due to an oligosaccharide such as glucose.

Tick vectors and their life cycles have been discussed by Davis (219, 220) who listed in the Americas *O. hermsi* Wheeler, Herms, and Meyer 1935 and *O. parkeri* Colley 1936 from the Western United States; *O. rudis* Karsch 1880 from Colombia, Venezuela, and Panama; *O. talaje* Guérin-Ménerville 1849 from the same area and also Argentina; and *O. turicata* Duges 1876 from the United States and Mexico, among the *Borrelia*-carrying ticks in the Western Hemisphere. Desportes and Campany (237) enumerated *O. tholozani* Laboulène and Méguin 1882 and other ticks of Asia Minor and Central Asia. Enigk and Grittner (257) presented a general survey of ticks and their biology.

Baker and Wharton (41) in their monograph suggested that borreliae evolved with Acarinae. This hypothesis implies that borreliae were primarily symbionts or parasites of ticks, specialized in *Ornithodoros* species by genetic evolution and adaptation, and invade mammals only by chance. This theory can be brought in accord with that of Nicolle and Anderson (520, 522) that ticks conserve and lice propagate borreliae, even though the latter authors believed that borreliae originated as parasites of small mammals, which does not seem plausible from today's vantage point.

The monographs of Baker and Wharton (41) and of Arthur (26) on ticks, that of Cooley and Kohls (200) on Argasidae in the Americas, the list by Hoogstraal of ticks in North Africa (371) and by Galouzo (290) in Central Asia, the review by Anastos (15) of Ixodides in the U.S.S.R., and numerous special communications of the group led by Geigy, Burgdorfer, and Aeschlimann on African ticks *(vide infra)*, together with the reviews by Nicolle *et al.* (529) and by Heisch (343), should be consulted for details.

Other and equally important reviews of *Ornithodoros* and tick-*Borrelia* relationships include that of Bohls (89), who listed *O. venezolensis* among the tick vectors in the Americas, and described their habits and habitats as follows. In the Western United States and in Texas, *Ornithodoros* like to establish themselves firmly in caverns, in Southwest Kansas in burrows of prairie dogs, in the State of Washington in owl burrows, and in Southwest Texas in rodent burrows. Domestic animals do not appear to be hosts of these ticks in the United States but *O. venezolensis* and *O. talaje* are often found in or near human habitations, *O. turicatae* in Texas sometimes under houses, and *O. hermsi* in or near summer cabins at relatively high altitudes, above 5,000 feet. Bohls pointed out that a tick species may be infested but does not have to cause human infection. Also, the tick population may be so lightly infested that samples collected from it may not reveal the presence of borreliae.

Baltazard and his group (53) observed different conditions in Asia and Africa. *O. erraticus* was found feeding on rodents in burrows. These authors listed studies on the so-called crocidurae subgroup of borreliae and discussed Central Asian strains. Cooley (199) stated that *O. erraticus* Lucas 1849 dwells in pig sties and burrows, and may have several hosts including frogs *(Bufo pantherinus)*. *O. moubata* Murray 1877 lives with man and domestic animals in Africa. *O. savignyi* Audouin 1826 in Africa and Asia keeps similar company. Not all authors agree, however, that *O. savignyi* is an effective carrier of borreliae. *O. cholodovskyi* Pavlovsky 1930 lives in Turkestan; *O. lahorensis* Neumann 1918 in

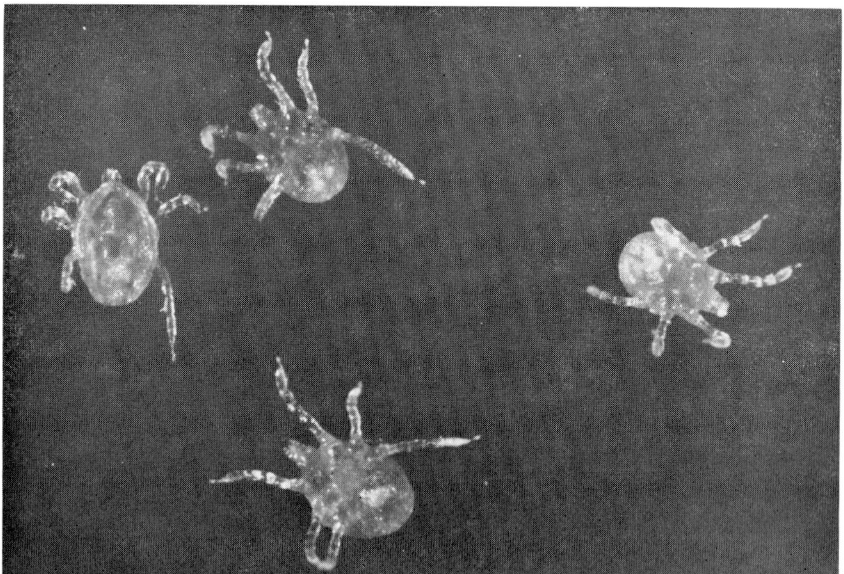

FIGURE 10. *Ornithodoros tartakovskyi,* nymphs. Photograph by Dr. T. C. Orihel.

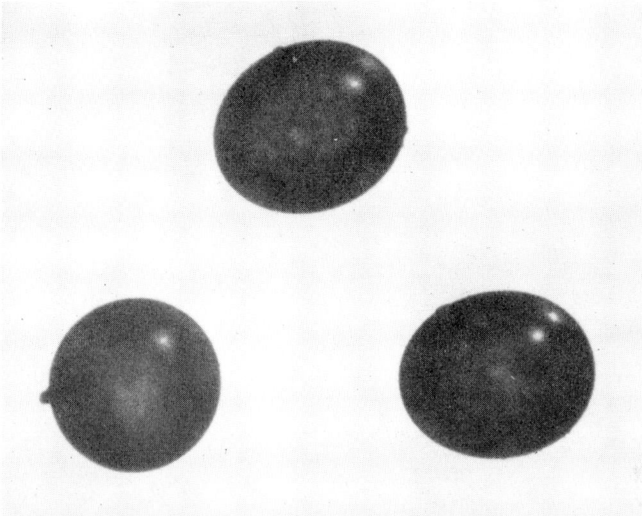

FIGURE 11. *Ornithodoros tartakovskyi* eggs.

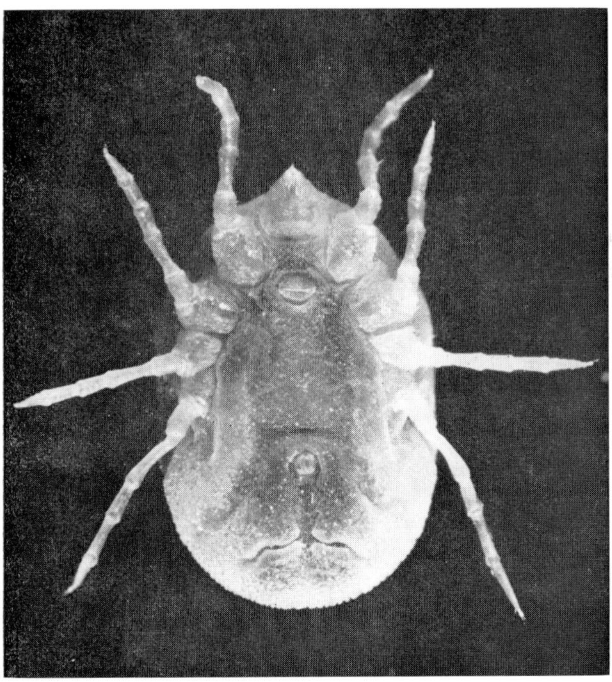

FIGURE 12. *Ornithodoros tartakovskyi,* adult femals, ventral view. Photograph by Dr. T. C. Orihel.

an area from India to Turkey and Palestine, with domestic and wild animals, as well as with man; *O. tartakovskyi* Olenev 1931 in Central Asia with *Tatera* and other animals; *O. tholozani* Laboulbène and Méguin 1882 (synonym *O. papillipes*) in Central Asia and Iran with man, camels, chickens, and in rodent burrows.

Hindle (365) pointed out that *B. normandii* may be identical to *B. hispanica* de Buen 1926; *B. sogdiana* Nicolle and Anderson 1928 and *B. uzbekistana* Picoul 1928 may be the same as *B. persica* Dshunkowsky 1913. He also identified the crocidurae Leger 1917 subgroup with *B. duttonii* Novy and Knapp 1906 which is contrary to serologic, epidemiologic, and clinical experience, if we speak in terms of species of *Borrelia* at all.

Davis (222) in his review maintained the theory of tick specificity but emphasized that numerous exemptions are possible, as *B. microti* being transmitted both by *O. lahorensis* and *O. canestrini* (236). He also pointed out the confusion existing with re-

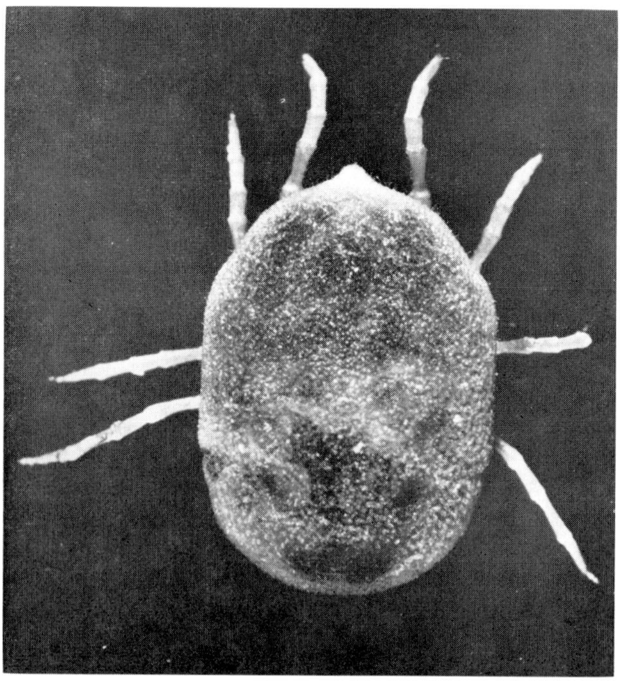

FIGURE 13. *Ornithodoros tartakovskyi,* adult female, dorsal view. Photograph by Dr. T. C. Orihel.

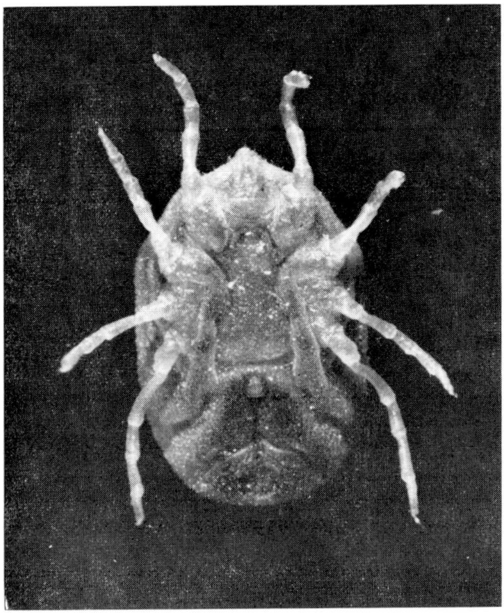

FIGURE 14. *Ornithodoros tartakovskyi,* male, ventral view. Photograph by Dr. T. C. Orihel.

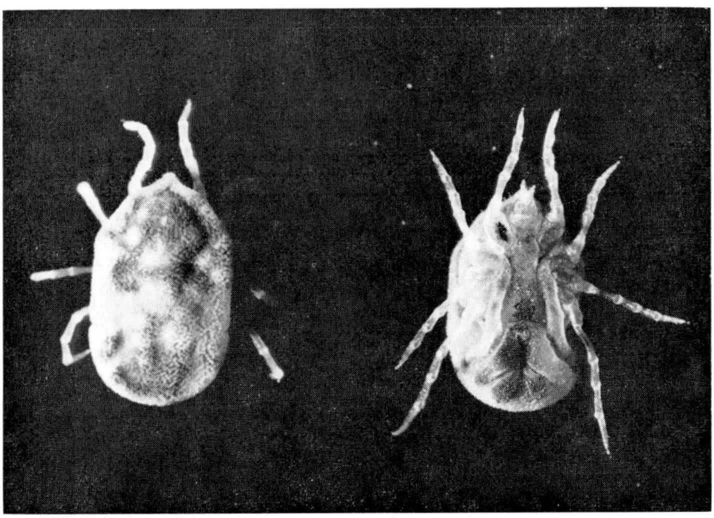

FIGURE 15. Dorsal *(left)* and ventral *(right)* view of *Ornithodoros tartakovskyi,* male.

spect to American ticks. *O. rudis* is synonymous with *O. venezolensis (O. venezuelensis)* and is the vector of *B. venezolensis* Brumpt 1921 and *B. neotropicalis* Bates and Saint-John 1922. *B. neotropicalis* has been reported also from Panama where it is transmitted by *O. rudis. O. talaje* bites animals but not man. Clark (182) believed that it transfers the infection only from animals to animals, whereas *O. rudis* takes part in the animal-vector-man-animal cycle. Davis also discussed the role of coxal fluid in the transmission of borreliae. Coxal fluid is expelled by the feeding tick as it becomes engorged with blood. It contains and transmits borreliae to the wound caused by the bite of the tick. Many ticks, like *O. turicata,* and particularly nymphs, do not expel coxal fluid but infect through their bite. This will be discussed in detail later.

Horsfall (374) added to the list of ticks carrying relapsing fever *O. brasiliensis* that harbors *B. brasiliensis, O. tholozani* as a carrier of *B. babylonensis, O. normandi* as a vector of *B. normandii,* and *O. dugesi* as a carrier of *B. dugesii.* It is doubtful, however, that *B. babylonensis* and *B. normandii* represent independent species. Horsfall emphasized that *O. erraticus* has two subspecies, namely, *O. erraticus erraticus,* the large form, the vector of *B. hispanica;* and *O. erraticus sonrai,* the small form, carrying members of the crocidurae subgroup. *O. e. erraticus* likes some moisture, *O. e. sonrai* dry burrows.

Nicolle and Anderson (524) stated that *Ornithodoros* have to be infected in the nymphal stage to become effective vectors.

Ornithodoros, therefore, may propagate borreliae from one generation to another. The borreliae may be transmitted to man and animals through the coxal fluid which contaminates the site of the insect bite, or, principally by young nymphs and in North American species also by adult ticks, through the salivary glands. The tick does not have to be injured, as does the louse, to transfer *Borrelia* to man or animals.

Observations on individual *Ornithodoros* and *Borrelia* species that are important from the medical point of view follow.

Specific Ticks and Borreliae

Ornithodoros moubata and Borrelia duttonii

Ornithodoros moubata, the eyeless tampan, has four subspecies, *O. compactus, O. apertus, O. porcinus,* and *O. porcinus domesti-*

cus (714, 715). It carries *B. duttonii.* Its principal homes are West and East Africa. Manson and Thornton (467) stated that the infection is severe, with many complications, in Europeans; severe but with few complications in the indigenous population. Moreover, these authors believed that several strains of *B. duttonii* may be carried by *O. moubata.* The organisms were described as 20 to 35 μ long, about 0.25 μ wide, with 5 to 9 spirals. Short and longer forms were common. Of 600 *O. moubata* ticks, 29% harbored borreliae. Dubois (247) also found different serotypes of *B. duttonii* in this tick.

Feng and Chung (270) could observe borreliae for a long time (11 days) in the stomach of *O. moubata* after a blood meal, but the borreliae appeared in the celomic fluid and in the salivary glands, neural ganglion, and coxal glands of the tick as early as within 6 hours. Multiplication of the borreliae took place in the organs and celomic cavity, by transverse division. No borreliae were seen by these authors in the Malpighian tubules or in the feces. The same writers stated later (271) that the central neural ganglion is the predilection site of *B. duttonii.* After long starvation, the borreliae may disappear from the coxal fluid and ovaries (428). The tick can fast long, even a year or more, and remain

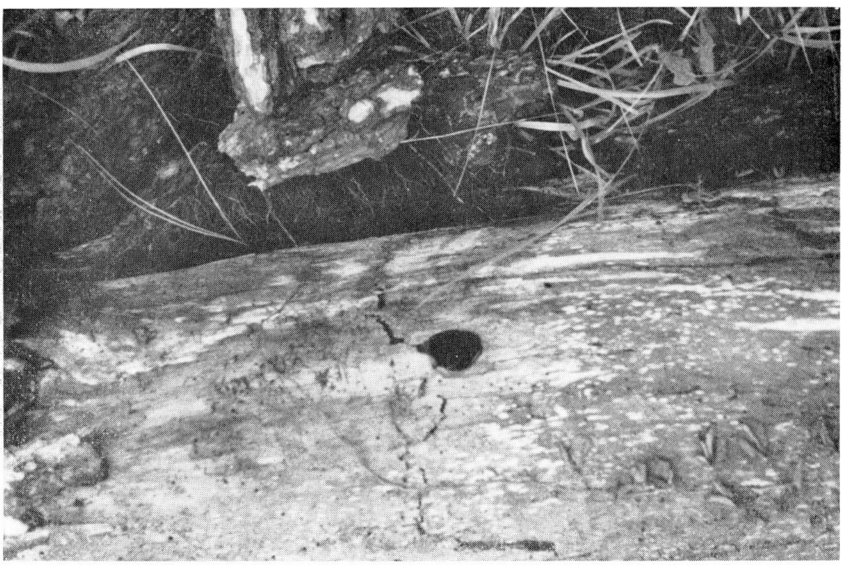

FIGURE 16. Holes in fallen trees, where *Ornithodoros turicata* were found.

alive. Adults usually feed every 6 weeks, nymphs every 2 to 3 weeks.

The subspecies of *O. moubata* usually prefer a single animal

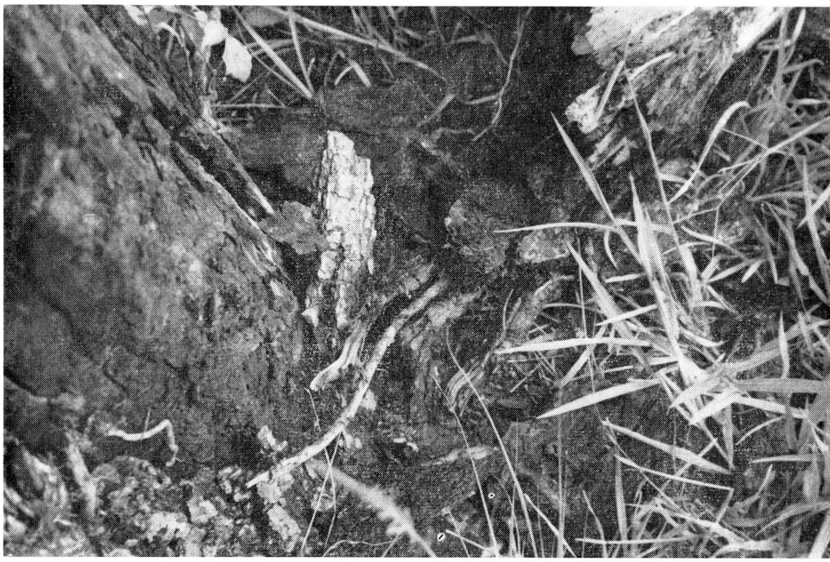

FIGURE 17. Rodent burrows harboring *Ornithodoros turicata.*

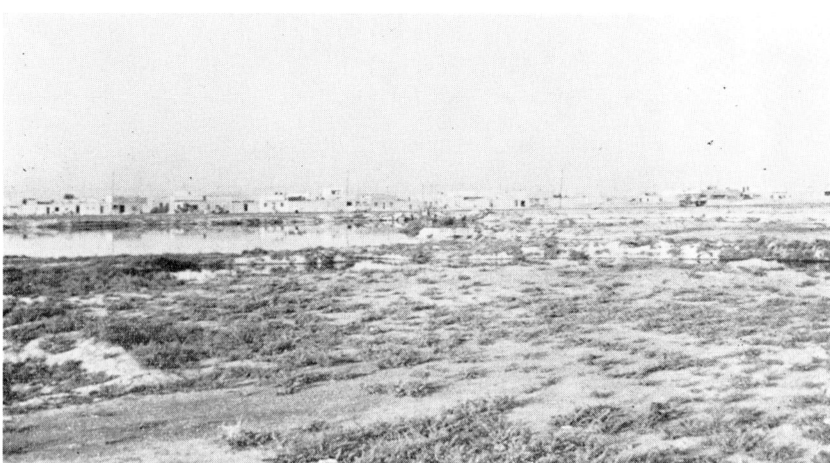

FIGURE 18. Semidesert in Asia, harboring *Ornithodoros erraticus* with small rodents.

host for their blood meal (309, 709). The blood meal lasts 20 to 30 minutes but the blood is digested very slowly. Precipitin tests showed its presence 7 months after feeding (721). The blood passes through the esophagus into the midgut and its diverticula which are relatively spacious and have quite elastic walls.

Molting takes place between meals. The life-span of *O. moubata* is 2 years, on the average. They withstand severe dehydration (110, 134).

Transovarian transmission of borreliae is the rule in *O. moubata*. Males may harbor *B. duttonii* in the genital organs but do not transfer them by the sexual act (313). Freshly fed females

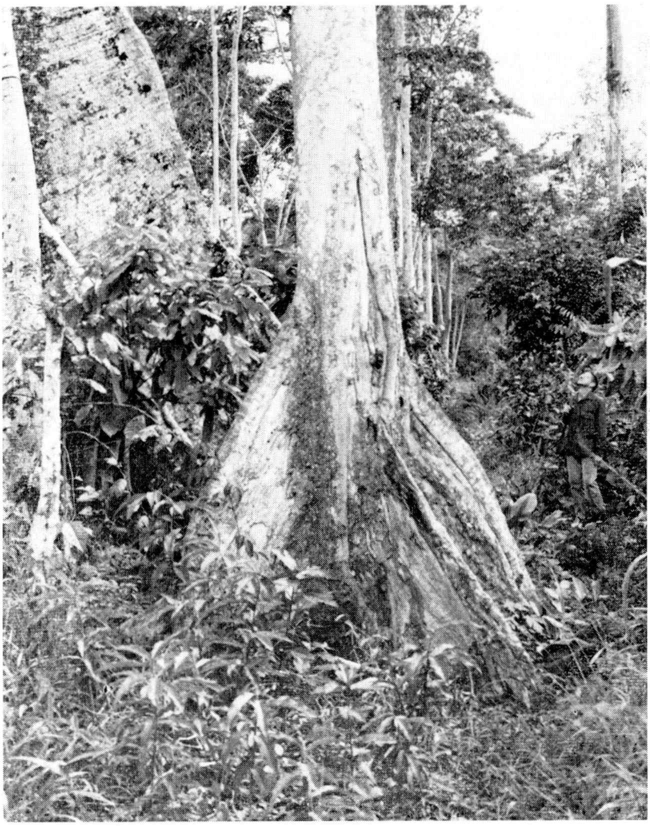

FIGURE 19. African forest with rodent burrows. Photograph by Dr. Clyde Jones.

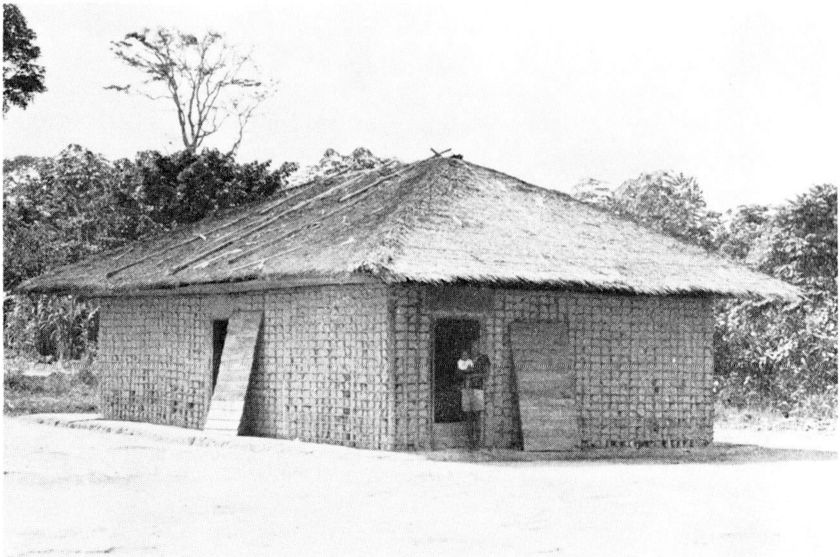

FIGURE 20. African hut in which *Ornithodoros moubata* thrives. Photograph by Dr. Clyde Jones.

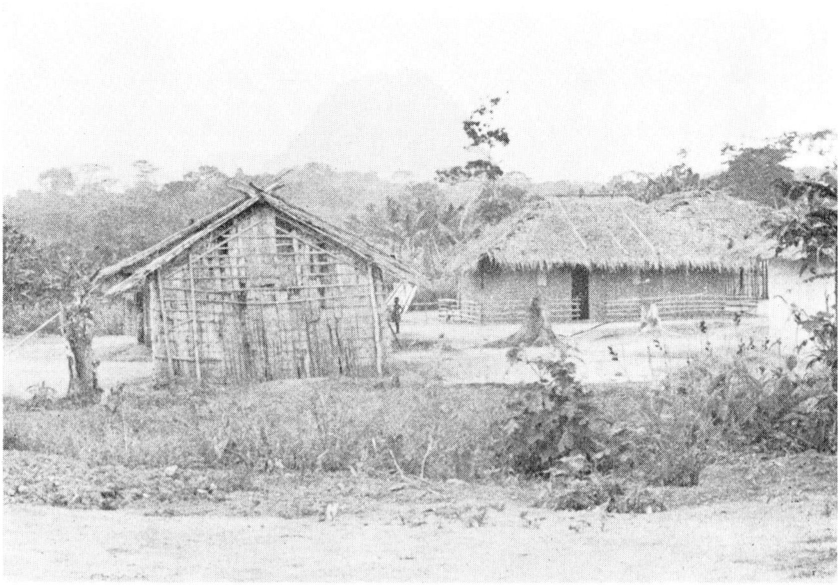

FIGURE 21. Huts with wooden walls *(foreground)* and clay walls *(back)* in Africa, where *Ornithodoros moubata* has been found. Photograph by Dr. Clyde Jones.

mate, burrow into the sand, and lay 30 to 80 eggs of about 0.6 mm diameter (303). The six-legged larvae hatch best at about 25° C. Six 8-legged nymphal stages follow, then the adult stage, within about 8 months. About 40 to 60% of the offspring are infected with *B. duttonii* (313). This proportion may vary, however, from one village to another, with an average of 15% (303). The salivary glands are irregularly infested in adults but contain many borreliae in the nymphs (699). Therefore, young adults and nymphs propagate the infection principally through their saliva, whereas adults spread it through the coxal fluid (302). The tick becomes infective 5 to 6 days after feeding on blood that contains *B. duttonii*. The first nymphal instar is the most effective transmitter also because of its rapid mobility. Geigy and Burgdorfer (129, 300, 301, 302, 306) demonstrated the efficiency of *O. moubata* in maintaining the infection without a vertebrate host.

O. moubata is found only in Africa but not in the dry desert,

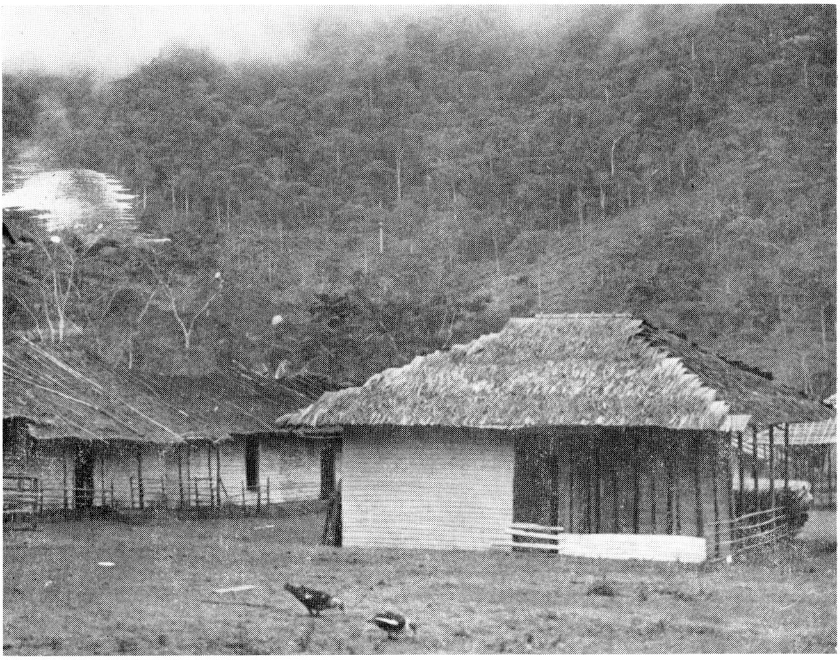

FIGURE 22. Huts in which man and fowl live together in Africa, where *Ornithodoros moubata* has been found. Photograph by Dr. Clyde Jones.

the rain forest, or above an altitude of 2,000 meters (6,600 ft.). *O. moubata* prefers fine loam on which African huts are built and in which man and fowl live together (712). *O. moubata* does not

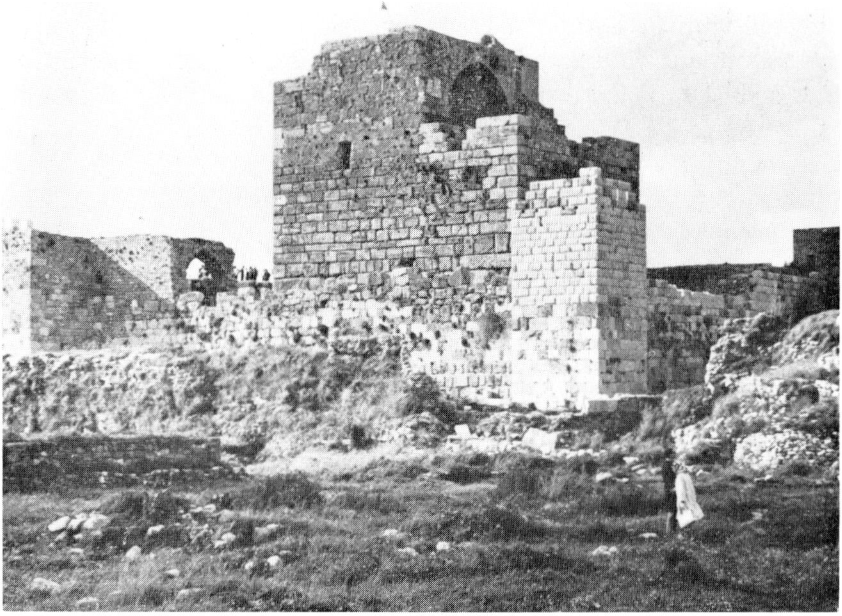

FIGURE 23. Ruins in the Mediterranean region where *Ornithodoros erraticus* was found.

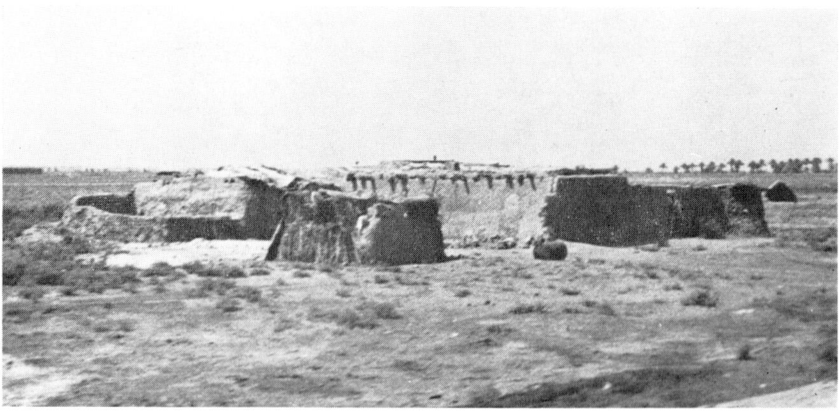

FIGURE 24. *Ornithodoros tholozani* was found in this building.

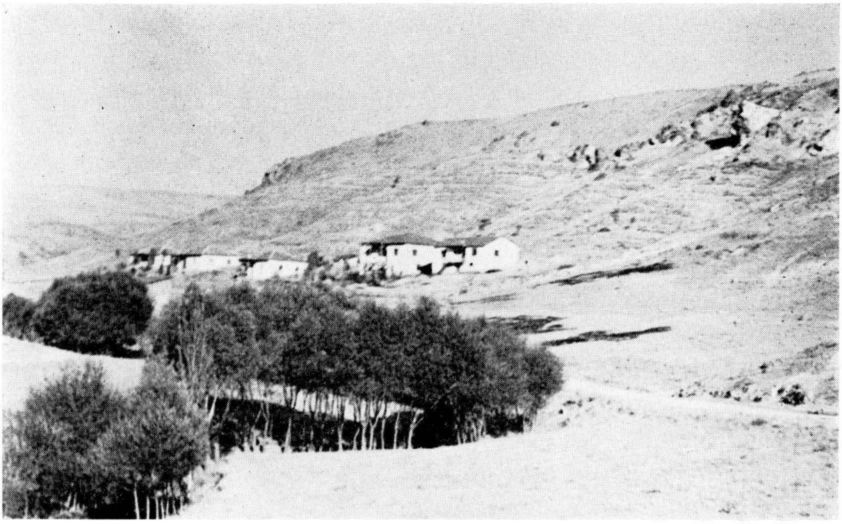

FIGURE 25. The home of *Ornithodoros tartakovskyi.*

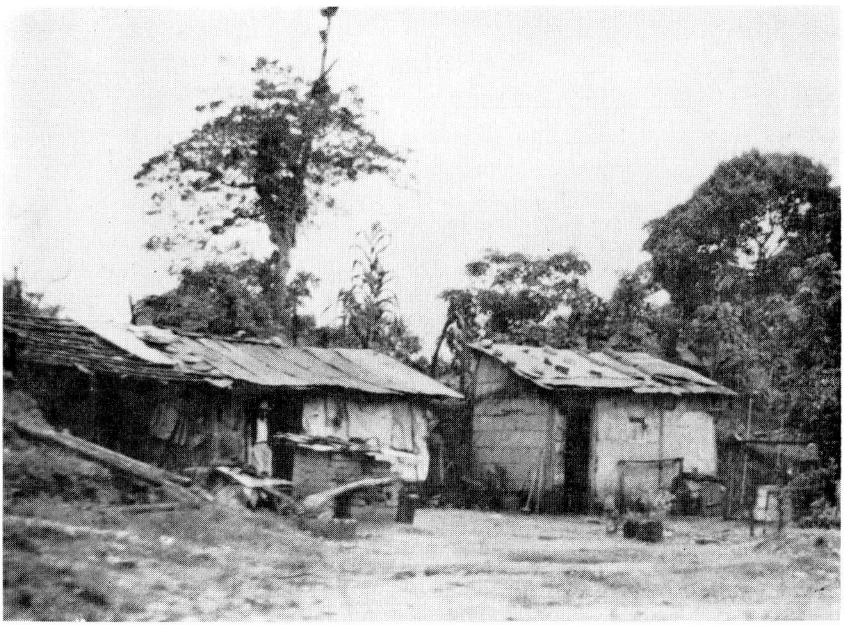

FIGURE 26. *Ornithodoros talaje*-infested building.

climb well, and likes to bury itself in the soil a few centimeters deep, particularly near dry places where people usually sit. It may be found in cracks, holes, and crevices of the mud floors and sometimes also in the grass walls. *O. moubata* appears to be domesticated but is still found in burrows of wart hogs, porcupines, hyenas, aardvarks *(Orycteropus)*, and bats (344). Walton (711) believed that its original hosts were these animals, and that it came to human habitations with hunters. This tick adapts itself easily to other hosts and may learn to bite cats, dogs, and pigs which, however, are not susceptible to *O. duttonii* infections.

O. moubata emerges from its hiding places after sunset. It is attracted to the bodies of people sleeping on the floor, and to fire. All stages, except eggs and larvae, take blood meals.

Details of the transmission of *B. duttonii* were worked out by Geigy and his co-workers (301, 302, 306, 311, 312) and others. Burgdorfer (129) observed that borreliae shorten from about 22 μ to 10 μ, gather at the stomach wall, and penetrate it. No borreliae are present in the stomach two weeks after the infective meal. The hemolymph of the tick sometimes harbors borreliae as early as the second day. Multiplication takes place in the celomic cavity. The coxal glands and the central ganglion may be invaded even on the third day, the Malpighian tubes somewhat later, but their lumina remain free from borreliae. There is a crossing of borreliae between the hemolymph and the organs for which it has predilection. The process of invasion of the *Ornithodoros* is slower at 20° than 30° C environmental temperature. Varma (699, 700) found the central ganglion infected in all instances, whereas the coxal glands harbored borreliae in 75%, and the Malpighian tubules in 25% of the examined ticks. Sarasin (622) believed that *B. duttonii* can enter any firm organ of *O. moubata* but that it lives always in intercellular spaces except in the oocysts. Aeschlimann (8) studied the transovarian transmission. *B. duttonii* enters oocysts early. The borreliae are located in the intercellular spaces but become intracellular after the tunica propria is formed.

Grün (327) observed that *O. moubata* did not acquire *B. duttonii* when this organism became nonpathogenic after numerous animal passages. The same strain of *O. moubata* could, however, transmit *B. hispanica*. Some loss of virulence of *B. duttonii* in the

5th generation of *O. moubata* was described by Aeschlimann (9). The transstadial and transovarian development, including the problem of filial variations in relation to the number of infective progenies, was summarized by Burgdorfer and Varma (130).

Colas-Belcour *et al.* (189) studied ticks from Madagascar which were not naturally infected and found that about 50% of these *O. moubata* will acquire *B. duttonii* if given a blood meal containing this *Borrelia.*

Further problems of the *O. moubata-B. duttonii*-animal-man relationship were investigated by several workers. Heisch and Grainiger (350) found that *O. moubata* living in rodent burrows is not a reservoir for human infection because of the rarity of contact between man and tick in the areas inhabited by wild rodents. Arboni (23) stated that *O. moubata* may live with guinea pigs, rabbits, pigeons, other fowl, and horses, but not uniformly with pigs. Fresh cattle, goat, and sheep serum killed *B. duttonii* but this activity of the serum was destroyed by heating. The origin and quality of the antibodies in these sera are open to question. Geigy and Mooser (305) studied wart hogs, the natural host of a variant of *O. moubata,* without being able to find proof of infection.

Geigy and Herbig (308) stated that *O. moubata* does not have a known and useful natural host. On the other hand, Walton (712) observed *O. moubata* in the Digo district of Kenya near the border of Tanganyika but only in houses that also sheltered fowl. The ticks harbored *B. duttonii* but human cases of infections were rare. Walton considered this an example of an animal reservoir without overspill into the human population. It is possible, however, that the human inhabitants had acquired immunity during undiagnosed episodes of infection in their childhood, or that the ticks preferred to feed on chickens. Schwetz (633) also found infected *O. moubata* but no borrelemia in human beings who lived in the same huts in various localities between Lake Kivu and Lake Albert in the Congo. He explained this as a state of immunity following past infection in the local inhabitants.

O. moubata is an effective vector. It was shown to be able to carry *B. hispanica* for many months in laboratory experiments (296) but not the East African strain of *B. recurrentis.* Baltazard *et al.* (54) had moderate success in transmitting *B. crocidurae* to it. *B. turicatae* lived in *O. moubata* in the laboratory for a long time but the tick did not transmit the *Borrelia*. Thus *O. moubata* appears to be carrying only *B. duttonii* in nature.

Ornithodoros erraticus erraticus and Borrelia hispanica

Ornithodoros erraticus erraticus or the "large" *O. erraticus* carries *Borrelia hispanica.*

Several strains of *B. hispanica* have been described. We believe, however, with Nicolle *et al.* (528), that both the so-called Moroccan and Mansourian (Bou Znika) strains are *B. hispanica,* as well as those labelled as Tripoli, Portuguese, Peloponese or Greek, and Normandian (South Tunisian) strain. Moreover, we include the atypical Syrian and Algerian strains (511, 625) also in this species.

The disease caused by *B. hispanica* is usually mild (230) whichever subtype is causing it. Exceptions are not rare, however.

According to Muñoz Cosin (510) *O. e. erraticus* is a nocturnal tick. It feeds for 15 to 20 minutes. It tolerates lack of food well even at 28° and 30° C if the humidity is high enough. *O. e. erraticus* apparently requires somewhat higher atmospheric moisture than does *O. moubata.* The borreliae are transmitted to the host after feeding, with the coxal fluid, but infection by the bite of the tick is also possible (277).

O. e. erraticus appears to have followed the route of the Moslem conquest, along the Mediterranean Littoral through North Africa to Spain. It established itself also in Portugal and Greece. The Moroccan strain was found in ticks in burrows of porcupines (230); others also in the dwellings of gerbils, hedgehogs, jackals, and wild rats (54); Muñoz Cosin (510) in addition to the foregoing observed the tick living with foxes, weasels *(Mustela vulgaris),* and pigs. It seems that pigs do not become infected with *B. hispanica* but may disseminate the tick. Neither is there an agreement that foxes are susceptible to *B. hispanica* infection. Baltazard (45) confirmed the findings of Nicolle and his coworkers in Tunisia, and isolated *B. hispanica* from wild rats, man, and *O. e. erraticus* in Casablanca. Delanoë (232) found hedgehogs infected, as well as young jackals. Older jackals appeared to have antibodies against *B. hispanica.* Young porcupines were also susceptible but grown animals had measurable antibodies (231). Similar results were observed in weasels (233). Wild rats were found infected in Greece (141). Nicolle and Anderson (527) examined closely the relationship of hogs to relapsing fever in North Africa. *B. hispanica* did not circulate in their blood. Even though they may act as host to *O. e. erraticus,* they did not appear to be important as animal reservoirs of relapsing fever. A survey of cave-dwelling bats in Spain (515) showed 4 susceptible species *(Miniopterus schreibersii, Myotis myotis, Rhinolophus euryale,* and *R. hipposideros).*

Mathis *et al.* (480) commented on the observation that tick-borne relapsing fever in Tropical Africa is due to *O. moubata* with the exception of Dakar, where *O. erraticus* was also found. Boiron (95, 96, 97) investigated this problem and found that 18.5% of the blood and 40% of the brain or spleen specimens from 512 rodents belonging to 9 species were infected. *Cricetomys gambinus* and *Rattus rattus alexandrinus* were most frequently infected, and *O. e. erraticus* was found on them. More cases were in modern Dakar than in the adjacent township of Medina. The number of rat burrows in the hard soil of Dakar was higher than in the light sandy soil of Medina. Also, *O. e. erraticus* appeared to find more feasible moist shelter in Dakar. Boiron also stated that hedgehogs and some reptiles may serve as hosts but man encounters *O. e. erraticus* easily in Dakar.

Not only *R. r. alexandrinus* in Dakar has been found to be an important reservoir but also other rats have been implicated, as the gray rat *(Ratus norvegicus)* in Casablanca (85) and in Algeria (373, 465). The role of the porcupine in Africa was more closely investigated by Nicolle *et al.* (530). They concluded that porcupines may be reservoirs of *B. hispanica* but live away from human habitation and roads and are, therefore, not an important source of human infection.

O. erraticus was found feeding on crabs when mammalian blood was not available. The crabs were resistant to borreliae and their blood remained free of them (50).

Jahnel (382) studied the fate of *B. hispanica* in hibernating dormice. The borreliae disappeared faster in the cold than at room temperature. If the animals were infected during hibernation, *B. hispanica* was recovered over longer periods than when the infection took place before hibernation.

B. hispanica, Tripoli strain, was maintained by Nicolle and Blaizot (531) through 12 rabbit passages without loss of virulence. Chorine and Colas-Belcour (167), however, found gradual diminishing of virulence after human passages, at a slower pace also in rodents. The incubation period also becomes longer.

Brumpt (123) described *B. babylonensis* from *O. asperus* which, however, was easily transmitted by *O. persica.* It caused many relapses in guinea pigs and the organisms in the blood were as numerous as in *B. hispanica* infections. *O. tholozani* and *O. erraticus* could not be infected with this strain. *O. coriaceus* (which does not transmit any known *Borrelia*) could not transmit it. This strain, unfortunately lost by now, may bc a variant or a transient organism, especially since *O. asperus* was shown to transmit *B. persica* in the laboratory. The geographical location of the finding of this *Borrelia* tips the balance in favor of *B. babylonensis* being a strain of *B. persica.*

Experimentally, *B. hispanica* has been transmitted to *Argas persicus, O. moubata, O. savignyi, O. tholozani, O. turicata, Haemaphysalis inermis, Pediculus humanus, Hemstopinus suis,* and *Xenopsylla cheopis* by Muñoz Cosin (510) and to *O. moubata* by Kudicke *et al.* (428). It was isolated from the dog tick *Rhipicephalus sanguineus* in Greece (141). Davis and Mavros (227) observed its survival in *O. nicollei* for 5 years and noted that it was transmitted to the F_1 generation in this tick. Baltazard *et al.* (54) transmitted *B. hispanica* by *O. savignyi, O. moubata,* and *Rhipicephalus sanguineus* in the laboratory. It appears that this *Borrelia* can be transmitted in the laboratory by many genera and species of insects. It is questionable if the same holds true in nature.

Ornithodoros erraticus sonrai and the "Crocidurae" Subgroup

Ornithodoros erraticus sonrai or the "small" *O. erraticus* is the vector of a group of borreliae that are only moderately or not at all pathogenic for man, but may cause disease in rodents (60, 480). The first member of the group, *B. crocidurae,* shows some cross-immunity with *B. duttonii* (525). Some experts consider *B. crocidurae* identical to *B. merionesi* and *B. microti,* whereas *B. dipodilli* of Kenya is regarded as a distinct strain (303). Baltazard *et al.* (53, 60) reported this group in Senegal, from the countries along the Southern Mediterranean, Iran, and East Africa. There is considerable disagreement concerning the status of the individual strains of the crocidurae subgroup. One of the principal reasons for the separation of this group was the difference in the tick vector. *B. crocidurae* was isolated from the wild shrew *(Crocidura stämpfii)* in Dakar by Leger in 1917. *B. crocidurae* is more virulent than the other members of the subgroup and often fatal for rats *(Cricetomys gambianus, Rattus rattus alexandrinus, Ratus norvegicus,* and *Arvicanthis sp.),* rarely for *Epimys, Rattus* and *Mus musculus* (478). Local people in Dakar appeared to be immune to *B. crocidurae* (481). Baltazard *et al.* (62) isolated it in Turkey, and found that this strain causes prolonged disease in guinea pigs but only weak or subclinical infections in man. Colas-Belcour (188) considered *B. crocidurae, B. microti,* and *B. merionesi* immunologically interrelated but different from *B. hispanica.* Dirk van Peenen (241) studied borreliae in *O. e. sonrai* that were found with Nile rats *(Arvicanthis niloticus)* by Davis and Hoogstraal in Egypt. Newborn rats and mice seem to be susceptible to *B. crocidurae* but adult guinea pigs are not. Some investigators (195, 303) emphasized that *O. e. erraticus* is not hospitable to *B. crocidurae* but that this organism was transmitted by the ovum to the F_1 generation of that tick subspecies. Vertebrates were infected during feeding, through the saliva of the infected tick. *O. e. erraticus* did not carry other members of the crocidurae subgroup.

B. merionesi was isolated in South Morocco by Baltazard. It was studied by Baltazard's group (see above) and was found to be different from *B. duttonii* and *B. hispanica.* It frequently caused fatality in rats and hamsters. Blanc and Maurice (84) found it nonpathogenic to man.

B. microti was isolated from *Microtus mistacinus* and from *Tatera indica,* as well as from rats and *Cricetulus migratorius* in Hessarak and other localities in Iran by Rafyi (592). This strain did not infect guinea pigs but caused some disease in man. Delpy (234) studied this organism in Iran and found 35% of *Tatera,* 14.8% of *Cricetulus,* and less than 12% of other rodents, such as *Nesokia, Mus,* and *Microtus,* infected with it. *Meriones shawi* also carried this *Borrelia.*

B. dipodilli was described by Heisch (342, 343) from pygmy gerbils *(Dipodillus gerbillus)* in Kenya. It was mildly pathogenic for rats, mice, monkeys, and young rabbits, but not for guinea pigs and man. Heisch believed that *B. dipodilli* is related to rodents in North Africa and the Middle East, and posed the question whether or not *B. duttonii* has evolved from it because of the belief that *B. duttonii* was originally a rodent-oriented *Borrelia*.

In laboratory experiments, *B. crocidurae* could be transmitted to the human louse but *P. humanus* did not transfer this organism to man (95, 98, 331). Monkeys have been found susceptible to *B. crocidurae* as well as to *B. merionesi* and *B. dipodilli*. The last (as well as *B. duttonii*) was able to infect the monkey louse, *Pedicinus longiceps,* and transmit the borreliae among nonhuman primates. The monkeys did not become seriously ill. This may point toward an additional life cycle of the members of the crocidurae subgroup. Ticks other than *O. e. sonrai* are not very hospitable to this group of borreliae (594). Therefore, adjustments, accommodation, and adaptation must have taken place before the present tick-reservoir of *B. duttonii* could develop, if the theory of Heisch is correct.

Ornithodoros tholozani (papillipes) and Borrelia persica

Ornithodoros tholozani (synonym: *Ornithodoros papillipes*) appears to be identical also to *O. crossi* which carries the Kashmir strain of *Borrelia*. It may have several subspecies. *O. tholozani* carries *B. persica*. *B. persica* was described by Dschunkowsky in 1913 (245). The domain of *O. tholozani* spreads from Lybia through Western Egypt, the Arab countries, Cyprus, and Turkey, to India and Central Asia. It is possible that *B. uzbekistanica* and *B. sogdiana* are variants of or identical to *B. persica* (444).

O. tholozani has one larval and 3 to 4 nymph stages. Each one of these stages feeds on a vertebrate at least once but the adults take a blood meal more often (691). Hereditary transmission is the rule (6, 42, 506, 691) but Bourgain (108, 580) failed to prove it. He suggested that the nymphs become infected during their blood meals.

O. tholozani lives for a long time. Bourgain (107, 108) reported that nymphs may live 5 years, if no food is available that is a prerequisite for molting; adults live about 7 years.

Adler *et al.* (5) and others showed that *B. persica* is transmitted by the bite of *O. tholozani* and not by the coxal fluid. Slavina (651) found 2% of ticks collected in their natural habitat infected with *B. persica*.

It appears that infected nymphs (108) and adult ticks (42) may lose borreliae during their lives, and the virulence of the strains may decrease in the ticks. Pirot and Bourgain (580) stated that infected ticks apparently die sooner than noninfected individuals. This problem should be further investigated since Balashov (42) saw an increased infection rate in successive tick generations, from 11 to 47%.

O. tholozani lives in caves and burrows of small animals in Central Asia in oases along the edges of the woodlands (563), and also with man. It was found in the huts of regimental followers in Qetta near the Afghan border (114), and collected in abandoned piggeries (691), often near fowl and camels.

Lice, especially those adapted to feeding on suckling rabbits, will take up *B. persica* (161).

O. tholozani has been infected artificially with *B. sogdiana* (21) but this experiment may have involved merely the transmission of the same strain or its variant. *B. recurrentis* can survive in *O. tholozani* (656) but lice fed on patients infected with *B. persica* do not transmit this organism. Rafyi and Maghami (594) were able to infect *O. tholozani* with *B. hispanica* and *B. microti*.

O. lahorensis has been thought of as a possible vector of *B. persica*. Pavlovskii (563) and others proved that this is not possible because *O. lahorensis* does not bite man and even though it acquires human-pathogenic borreliae by feeding on rodents in the laboratory, the borreliae die off in it rather quickly.

Babudieri (36) encountered two possibly distinct strains of *B. persica* in Jordan. One, the rural form, caused disease in sheepherders, migrants, road builders, and other persons who rest in caves with dry and sandy floors harboring *O. coniceps*. The peak number of infections was in the winter. The other, the urban form, appeared in badly maintained and ventilated houses with earthen floors. The greatest number of infections was observed in the summer. Babudieri believed that *O. tholozani* is the vector in urban areas, where domestic rats could serve as a reservoir of the infection. It is still being debated, however, whether *O. coniceps* is a vector of borreliae *(vide infra)*.

Ornithodoros tartakovskyi* and *Borrelia latyschewii

Sofiev (655) described *Borrelia latyschewii* from *Ornithodoros tartakovskyi*. This *Borrelia* was isolated from gerbils (*Rhombomys opimus* and *Gerbillus eversmanni*) as well as from *O. tartakovskyi* caught in burrows of rodents. It causes mild disease in man, often only a one-day fever, and one or two attacks in mice but not in rats, guinea pigs, and dogs. The number of borreliae is low in the blood even after successful infection. Sofiev and Leitman (656), analyzing tick- and louse-borne relapsing fever in Central Asia, pointed out that this *Borrelia* cannot be transmitted by lice to man in that region, nor can *O. tartakovskyi* propagate *B. recurrentis*. The latter *Borrelia* will, however, survive in *O. tartakovskyi* for 4 months.

Baltazard *et al.* (55) isolated *B. latyschewii* from *O. tartakovskyi* in Iran, near Meshed. This strain did not infect adult guinea pigs which is unusual in Old World tick-borne borreliae. The organism was slightly pathogenic for man but was not found in nature in rodents with which the tick lived. It appeared to prefer the burrows of merions and other wild rodents, tortoises, lizards, and toads. Wild rodents such as *Meriones, Microtus,* and *Rhombomys* could be infected in the laboratory.

O. tartakovskyi exudes coxal fluid some time after it has left the host on which it fed. This, perhaps, explains the small numbers of borreliae transmitted into the animal by the bite of the tick.

The natural reservoirs of the Central Asian and the Caucasian parts of the U.S.S.R. were studied by Pavlovskii (565). *Dryomys nitedullus,* a small, widely distributed rodent, is readily infected with borreliae and carries them for a month or longer. The principal foci were not associated with forests but with oases along the base of the mountains. Petrishcheva (571) investigated the duration of natural foci in Turkmenia. Not only *O. tartakovskyi* but also *O. tholozani* and *O. neerensis* were found. Caves inhabited by *Hystrix hirsutirostis* were studied but a change of the inhabitants of the burrows did not reduce the danger of infection for man. Of 13 foci, 8 were active 16 to 19 years, 2 for 21 to 29 years, and 3 for 30 years. This bears witness to frequent and sustained transmission cycles. Chickens, pigeons, gold fish, and 19 bird and reptile species were found resistant to *B. latyschewii* and *B. persica* in the same area (496). No borreliae were found in 1,144 reptiles caught in homes. Thus, reptiles cannot be considered a reservoir of Central Asian tick-borne relapsing fever borreliae.

O. tartakovskyi intrudes into animal sheds, cattle serving as a source of its blood meals. It may also invade floors and the lower parts of walls, hiding in cracks, holes, and crevices. Moreover, when new lands are being opened for agriculture, people may come into contact with *Borrelia*-carrying ticks, and the cycle tick-rodent-tick may be extended to tick-rodent-tick-man-tick-man-(rodent)-tick.

Ornithodoros neerensis is also supposed to carry *B. latyschewii* (566, 587). It is not known if the two tick strains are identical or related.

Orinthodoros verrucosus and Borrelia caucasica

Ornithodoros verrucosus, the vector of *Borrelia caucasica,* lives in burrows of merions *(Meriones erythrourus caucasicus), Apodemus sylvaticus,* and *Mus musculus.* The disease in man may be severe and consist of 10 to 15 relapses within 3 months. Chubaryan (171) found jerboas *(Alactaga elater, A. williamsi)* susceptible to the infection. Laboratory rodents acquire mild disease or are only slightly susceptible to this *Borrelia.* Guinea pigs develop several attacks. To the knowledge of this author, *B. armenica* has not yet been studied outside the U.S.S.R.

Ornithodoros zumpti and Borrelia tillae

Geigy (303), when considering *Borrelia tillae,* regarded it as a phylogenetic problem. It may have evolved from human-borne *B. duttonii* by progressive specialization because *O. moubata* does not feed on domestic rodents, and wild rodents are resistant to *B. duttonii.*

Zumpt (748) described the tick vector in 1959. Zumpt and Organ (749) reported on *Borrelia tillae* isolated from *O. zumpti* Heisch and Guggisberg living in holes of the South African field vlei rat *(Otomys saundersiae).* White mice and the multimammalian rat *(Rattus natalensis)* are highly susceptible to the infection. Patas monkeys *(Erythrocebus patas)* and adult guinea pigs, as well as some rabbits, were refractory to the infection. Geigy and Aeschlimann (305) succeeded in transmitting *B. tillae* to *O. moubata* but serologic tests and electron microscopic studies showed that *B. tillae* is not indentical to *B. duttonii*. Moreover, *B. tillae* was not pathogenic for white rats, hamsters, and merions. On further investigation, *B. tillae* was isolated also from the brains of the four-striped rat *(Rhabdomys pumilio)* and *R. natalensis*. Heisch and Harvey (354) confirmed these findings. One may expect further developments in the study of this interesting *Borrelia*.

Relapsing Fever Vectors and Borreliae in the Americas

Calero (137) surmised that the American relapsing fever strains are tick-adapted *B. recurrentis*. Brumpt (118) believed, however, that American borreliae did not become tick-borne after the Spanish Conquest or after the settlement of the West commenced when louse-borne relapsing fever was introduced. Tick-borne borreliae were probably already present in the western mountain ranges and lands when the first immigrants arrived. Kemp *et al.* (407), Wynns and Beck (741), Beck (69), Wheeler (727), Davis (271, 218), and others gave detailed accounts of the borreliae and their vectors in the Americas.

Ornithodoros turicata and Borrelia turicatae

Ornithodoros turicata Dugés 1876 is the vector of *Borrelia turicatae* Brumpt 1933. Kemp et al. (406) observed that larvae and nymphs feed 10 to 30 minutes, adults for hours and even for two days. The borreliae are transferred by the bite of this tick. Coxal fluid is secreted after meals but does not contain borreliae. *O. turicata* is easily infected with *B. turicatae*. Practically all adults carry it and propagate the *Borrelia* at least to the F_5 generation (221). Francis (278, 279) observed that starving *O. turicata* may survive for 5 years.

O. turicata has been found in Canada, the Western United States as far east as Kansas, in Mexico, and in South America. Caves, especially those which are entered by goats and sheep, and burrows of redents, such as those of field mice in Central Mexico (483), and burrows of owls and snakes are the habitats of *O. turicata*. It is found under houses in Texas (89) and it is becoming domesticated in Mexican huts and animal barns.

The central ganglion of the tick is not as hospitable to *B. turicatae* as it is to *B. duttonii.*

Brumpt and Brumpt (124) and Mazzotti (483) demonstrated that mice, rats, guinea pigs, cotton rats, rabbits, pigs, dogs, cats, and foxes can be infected with *B. turicatae* in the laboratory but not hedgehogs and dormice. The virulence for guinea pigs is low.

O. turicata cannot transmit *B. duttonii, B. venezolensis* (118), or *B. dugesii* Mazzotti 1949 (228).

Ornithodoros parkeri and Borrelia parkerii

Ornithodoros parkeri Cooley 1936 transmits *Borrelia parkerii* Davis 1942. It lives in the western region of Canada and the United States but not in Mexico, in caves and burrows inhabited by ground squirrels, prairie dogs, and burrowing owls (384). It only infrequently encounters man. The infection is transmitted by the bite of the tick because coxal fluid is excreted only after feeding. Rafyi *et al.* (593) described a variant of *O. parkeri* that was found on the Hastings Reservation in Monterey County, California. The *Borrelia* harbored by this variant differed antigenically from the type strain.

O. parkeri can be infested with *B. turicatae* but not with *B. venezolensis* in the laboratory (485).

Ornithodoros hermsi and Borrelia hermsii

Ornithodoros hermsi Wheeler, Herms, and Meyer 1935 was described in 1935, together with the *Borrelia* strain carried by it (730). It was found in the Californian mountains at an altitude between 5,000 and 8,000 ft, but human cases of borreliosis were discovered also at 3,000 ft. It is a disease acquired by persons entering newly opened wooden summer cottages which are frequented (when empty) by wild rodents such as *Tamiasciurus douglasii* and *Eutamias* that often carry this tick in their fur (358).

B. hermsii has been studied extensively by Wheeler (727, 728, 729). It is transmitted with the eggs but less than 2% of them are infested. *O. hermsi* does not extrude feces or coxal fluid during feeding. Its bite is infective. When mammalian blood is not available, *O. hermsi* may feed on other ticks. Mice and monkeys can be infected with *B. hermsii* (727). Three days after a meal on an infected rodent or man, the celomic cavity becomes invaded, and the central ganglion by the 10th day (728, 729). Longanecker (458) found *O. hermsi* in dead trees ("snags") at an altitude of 6,000 to 8,000 ft. Of 39 batches of *O. hermsi,* 18 infected mice, rats, and chipmunks.

Ornithodoros talaje and its Borreliae

Ornithodoros talaje Guérin-Méneville 1848 probably has substrains. It is principally a Central and South American tick, found on the West Coast of the Americas and in Argentina. Bates *et al.* (68) observed *O. talaje* in the Arriján area of Panama. Human infections were present there. Rats, mice, and *Macaca mulatta* monkeys could be infected by the bite of *O. talaje.* Dunn and Clark (248) described natural infections in marmoset monkeys *(Sanguinus geoffroyi), Cebus capucinus,* opossums *(Didelphis marsupialis etensis),* armadillos *(Dasypus novemcinctus fenestratus),* cattle, and in a horse. *O. talaje* transfers borreliae rather from animal to animal than from animal to man (182, 222) even though it often appears near human habitats (89). It attaches itself to opossums and other animals that prowl around horses and cattle tied to bush fence posts in which *O. talaje* then finds a home. It may also crawl under houses.

Vampire bats and *Triatoma* bugs may acquire this *Borrelia* but do not transmit it to other animals. Some strains of *O. talaje* do not bite man (222, 577). The *Borrelia* transmitted by *O. talaje* has not yet been named because it was believed that it is identical to that from *O. rudis.* Matters became complicated when Calero (137) stated that *B. neotropicalis* is a variety of *B. recurrentis* carried by *O. venezolensis* (synonym: *O. rudis)* as well as by *O. talaje.* Mazzotti (484, 485) found incongruities between the bionomics of *O. venezolensis* and *O. talaje* on one hand, and *B. venezolensis* on the other hand. Davis (225) stated that *O. dugesi* is a possible alternate host of *B. talaje,* and described *B. mazzottii sp.nov.* from *O. talaje* from Mexico and Guatemala that transmitted this *Borrelia* regularly, and *O. dugesi* weakly and in a fleeting way. *O. talaje* from other areas (Panama) did not transmit *B. mazzottii,* nor did *O. venezolensis, O. turicata* from Mexico, and some other ticks. There was no transovarian passage in *O. talaje* carrying this *Borrelia.* Guinea pigs and young rabbits were refractory to it. Considering further that *B. venezolensis* (synonyms: *B. venezuelensis* Brumpt 1924, *B. neotropicalis* Bates and Saint John 1922) is present in *O. rudis* Karsch 1880 (synonyms: *O. venezuelensis* Brumpt 1921 and *O. venezolensis)* in approximately the same area, and that the differentiation of borreliae by immunologic and serologic means is most difficult, one could assume that *O. talaje* carried *B. mazzottii* and in addition a hitherto unnamed *Borrelia,* the vector being perhaps a subspecies of *O. talaje.* Further investigation of this problem is certainly indicated and, until such studies are carried out, one has to keep an open mind.

Ornithodoros venezolensis and Borrelia venezolensis

The synonyms were discussed under *O. talaje,* which is said to be able to carry also *B. venezolensis.* Pifano (573) found this tick in Venezuela and in Mérida on the Yucatán (Mexico). A "related" tick was discovered in Yayacuy. The tick acquired the habits of a bed-bug, and became domesticated. Rats and mice on which the tick was fed developed borrelemia. The *Borrelia* was neurotropic. No animal reservoir was found. The ticks appeared to feed only on man, as shown by precipitin tests with sera against various animal blood. Osorno Mesa (558) found *O. venezolensis* in Santander, Colombia, and suspected that human cases may exist there. Anduze (18) collected *O. venezolensis* in the Mérida area of Venezuela at an elevation between 1,600 to 5,000 feet. The human relapsing fever caused by its bite was severe. León and León (443) found the vector in Esmeraldes, Colombia, and varying clinical pictures of the disease. They suspected birds and wild rodents as the reservoir. Mazzotti (484) believed that *B. venezolensis* is the causative agent of relapsing fever in Panama, Colombia, and Venezuela, that *O. talaje* and *O. venezolensis* carry it, but perhaps that the strains are diffenent.

Other Borreliae

Ornithodoros brasiliensis Argão-Beaurepaire 1923 carries *Borrelia brasiliensis* Davis 1952 (224). This tick has one larval and 4 to 7 nymph stages before the adult emerges. It is able to feed two days after moulting. Davis was the first to rear these ticks in the laboratory. Little information is available about the disease caused by *B. brasiliensis* and the ecology of the ticks. It appears, however, that *B. brasiliensis* can be transmitted to mice and guinea pigs.

Heisch (345) described *Ornithodoros graingeri,* the vector of *B. graingeri* Heisch 1953 in Kenya. It caused disease in man, with slight neurotropism. The illness was mild in rats and mice. Guinea pigs, young rabbits, and monkeys were not susceptible.

Garnham (293) reported a *Borrelia* from a grivet monkey.

Carley and Pope (144) described *Borrelia queenslandica* from *Rattus villosus* in Australia. It caused relapses in mice and rats. Guinea pigs and chickens were not susceptible. This *Borrelia* could be carried in the laboratory in fertilized chick embryos. It was not transmitted by *O. gurneyi,* the only *Ornithodoros* species in the area where the organism was isolated.

Further data are not available on these borreliae.

Other Ornithodoros

Ornithodoros coniceps Canestrini 1890 was considered a possible vector of borreliae but Chagin and Diatlov (151) demonstrated that it is not infected in nature. However, about 2 to 3% of these ticks will take up *B. persica* when fed on infected animals, and will transmit this *Borrelia* to about 10% of the guinea pigs on which they are fed at a later date. Ovarian transmission has also been observed.

Ornithodoros lahorensis Neumann 1908, which was said to be a vector, was unable to transmit Central Asian borreliae in the hands of Pavlovskii and Kuzima (567). *O. lahorensis* is common in the stone walls of old caravanserais, in cracks of wooden buildings, and in sheep stalls. Perhaps it lives also with rodents in their burrows (584).

Ornithodoros foleyi Parot 1928 (synonym: *O. franchinii)* was considered a vector of *B. hispanica* in Lybia where two war-time louse-borne epidemics raged. Colas-Belcour and Vervent (191) were unable to prove that it plays a role in the propagation of relapsing fever.

Ornithodoros savignyi Audouin 1827 has been observed from Timbuktoo to Ceylon. It has never been found to be infected in nature although it takes up *B. duttonii* and *B. hispanica* in the laboratory (121). Considerable research has been devoted to this tick which lives outdoors, especially in places where camels, sheep, and other livestock rest. The reason is that it appears in areas where relapsing fever is present but generally accepted tick vectors are scarce, sporadic, or have not yet been found. One of these countries is Somaliland. Moise (497) suspected but did not prove that *O. savignyi* is an effective *Borrelia* vector. Kirk (410) could not transmit *B. recurrentis* to it in Abyssinia. Walton (710) showed that *O. savignyi* is a pure field tick. Lovett (461) in Somaliland found *O. moubata* to be a potent vector, but still believed that *O. savignyi* may participate in the dissemination of relapsing fever. Anderson (16) pointed out that *O. moubata* lives mostly indoors and has much more intimate contact with man so that it must be a much more effective vector.

Ornithodoros canestrini Birula 1845 was investigated as a possible vector of borreliosis by Delpy *et al.* (236) in Iran but neither *B. persica* nor *B. microti,* the borreliae of Iran, could be transmitted by this tick in animal experiments.

Unusual Vectors

A number of arthropods other than human lice and *Ornithodoros* have been considered as possible vectors of human relapsing fever. Bedbugs *(Cimex lectularis)* are the first in importance among these.

Rosenholz (611) surveyed the literature and in his own experiments found *B. duttonii* in the gut of bedbugs for 5 days after feeding, but borreliae did not find their way into the celomic cavity in all the bugs that were fed. *B. duttonii* survived for about 2 months in those that were successfully infested. Chung (172), studying an outbreak of epidemic relapsing fever in an orphanage in Peiping, stated that bedbugs may acquire *B. recurrentis* but the organism vanishes from their blood in one day. Furthermore, Chung and Feng (178) concluded from the results of their experiments that bedbugs, like lice, have to be crushed to transmit the infection. Francis (278) succeeded in transmitting *B. turicatae* by *C. lectularis.* Bonné (100) stated that while bedbugs and *Melophagus ovinus* can harbor borreliae for about 2 days after feeding, they do not transmit the organisms to mammals. Blanc *et al.* (82) observed considerable differences in the survival time of borreliae in bedbugs according to the microbial strain employed in the experiment. *B. hispanica* could be detected for 2 days, *B. persica* for 3 to 48, *B. duttonii* for 150, and *B. merionesi* for more than 200 days after infestation. The virulence of the borreliae did not diminish during their sojourn in the bedbug. Weyer and Moser (726) were able to preserve *B. recurrentis* and *B. hispanica* in frozen bedbugs.

The South American *Cimex rotundatus* was considered a possible vector of *B. venezolensis* by Pino-Pou (577).

The dog tick, *Rhipicephalus sanguineus,* has been another object of numerous querries. Sergent (637) found this insect, infected, on a dog belonging to a patient with relapsing fever in North Africa. Sergent (639) later reviewed the literature on this subject. Bonné (100) observed infected larvae. When the infective meal took place during the nymph stages, the adult *R. sanguineus* carried borreliae for about 3 months.

Members of the tick genus *Argas* are transmitting fowl borreliosis. It is natural that their relationship to human relapsing fever has also been investigated. Bonné (100) was unable to transmit African borreliae by *Argas reflexus.* Harold (337) asserted that *Argas persicus* does not bite man and is, therefore, not a probable vector of human relapsing fever.

The tropical rat mite *(Liponyssus nagayoi)* was studied by Omori (554). It transmitted *B. duttonii* from mouse to mouse for 12 days after the infective blood meal. Its feces and ova remained free from borreliae.

Fränkel (280) attempted to transmit epidemic relapsing fever from man to man by the stable fly *(Stomoxys calcitrans).* This fly, as many other biting insects, is able to harbor live borreliae in its gut for a few days but cannot transfer the organisms to man.

It is possible to paraphrase an axiom by saying that several borreliae may be looking for a vector, and several vectors for feasible hosts. Potential rodent reservoirs without active carriers of borreliae exist in several parts of the world. Huang (375), for instance, enumerated *Microtus mandarinus, Cricetus triton, C. barabensis, Micromys minutus,* and *Apodemus agrarius,* rodents living in the Yang-tse Valley in China, which represent such a potential reservoir. The disease is absent, however, principally because of the lack of an efficient and infected tick vector.

Portals of Entry

Transmission of borreliae takes place most often during the feeding of anthropophilic vectors of human pathogenic *Borrelia*.

During gestation, borreliae seem to be transmitted from the blood of the mother to the fetus (19), but the organisms are not transmitted through the milk to the offspring (292, 602). Infection may be acquired from the nursing mother, however, through mucous membranes (73). Menstrual blood also carries *Borrelia* (116). Skin excoriations as well as intact mucosal membranes may serve as portals of entry (54, 107, 364). Chung (174, 175) in China, observed that human urine and prostatic fluid may harbor borreliae. He was able to transmit the organisms to susceptible animals in the laboratory.

Laboratory infections have been described as having originated with human clotted blood kept for six days at room temperature (464), infected monkey blood (642), blood from the vein of a patient which squirted into the nose of a technician (429), and in one case, infection occurred in a laboratory worker who accidentally splashed patient's blood into his eyes and in another who was sprayed accidentally with placental blood (462). A classical example of a laboratory infection is that of an entomologist who was contaminated with the blood of a squirrel he was dissecting (442). Borreliae may be transmitted also with blood transfusions (596, 716). These are rare exceptions, however, and the classical route is infection by a feeding human louse or *Ornithodoros*.

Attempts to Classify Borreliae According to Response of Experimental Animals

The reader may have experienced considerable difficulties in perusing the preceding pages when attempting to sort out the various hosts or when sifting out the responses of experimental animals in the laboratory to infections with the different *Borrelia* strains. This author has to admit that the study of many of the individual reports quoted in this monograph was not always an easy task, for details of technics, of the mode of infection, the age and condition of the animals including their stock were not always made clear in some writings on this subject. The re-testing of many data is still a prerequisite for the formation of a clearer picture of the parasite-host relationship under laboratory conditions. This can be done by checking available reports by experimenting with accessible *Borrelia* strains and standardized methods. A critical evaluation of the procedures hitherto employed needs to be programmed by keeping in sight two goals: first, the ability of the vector to infect a given animal species. The results of such investigations will help to delineate the animal reservoir, the possible formation of biotopes, and therewith, assist in obtaining information useful from the epidemiologic point of view. Secondly, the question has to be answered whether a *Borrelia* separated from its vector and administered to a laboratory animal will or will not cause signs and symptoms valuable for the laboratory diagnosis of the strain.

Transmission by vectors has been discussed in the foregoing chapters, and will be analyzed again in the portion of this monograph dealing with epidemiology. At this point we are concerned with the susceptibility of laboratory animals, and with the possibility of their use in the classification of *Borrelia.*

Mice have been used for a long time in experimental borreliosis.

They are small, easily maintained, and usually on hand in larger laboratories. There is, however, the question of the route of inoculation, and the age and strain of the mice. Gray (322), for instance, stated that young mice are more susceptible to *B. duttonii.* Kemp *et al.* (406) found that mice are easily infected with North American borreliae. Wolman and Wolman (736) confirmed the susceptibility of mice to *B. recurrentis.* Coghill and Gambles (186) were able to produce short-term disease in mice by inoculating them with the blood or brain from patients in whom *B. recurrentis* could not be found by other methods in the peripheral circulation. Baltazard and his group (46, 59, 60, 61) emphasized the feeble but very constant susceptibility of mice to *B. recurrentis* and other borreliae. Baltazard (47) also demonstrated that the time of borrelemia in mice could be prolonged by splenectomy from the usual 3 days to a longer period. Kroó (425) emphasized that the virulence for mice varies with the strain of the *Borrelia* and with the relapse from which the infective material was collected. Durieux and Boiron (249), in their studies of relapsing fever in Dakar, used mice as indicators for their survey of the occurrence of borreliae in naturally infected animals, injecting the blood of such animals into laboratory mice.

Geigy and Aeschlimann (300, 305) showed that *B. duttonii* causes more persistent infection in mice than *B. recurrentis.* Sergent (638) reported that mice become ill 24 hours after inoculation with *B. hispanica* but recover after a short period.

Young mice were preferred and recommended by Geigy and others (300, 305, 662, 663) for laboratory experiments with borreliae. Guggenheim and Halevi (329) demonstrated that thiamin-deficient mice become more seriously ill than well-nourished mice when infected with borreliae.

Baltazard *et al.* (46, 59) found the response of adult rats to *B. recurrentis* somewhat variable even after splenectomy, but the borreliae were more pathogenic than they were for mice. Newborn rats became consistently infected, and the borreliae circulated longer in their blood than in the blood of mice according to these investigators (48, 99) who also preferred rats to mice because of their size and the ease with which they can be handled. Rats usually survive the infection, even though they may appear ill. Geigy and Aeschlimann (305) observed that *B. duttonii* is pathogenic but somewhat less for rats than for mice. Kalajew (393) found that splenectomized rats harbor in their circulation enormous numbers of borreliae with a long period of survival of these organisms in the brain. Rats are highly susceptible to the American strains of *Borrelia* (406, 407).

Rabbits appear more difficult to infect. Nicolle and Blaizot (532) had to inject large numbers of *B. recurrentis* intravenously to observe borrelemia lasting 2 days. Sergent (638), using *B. hispanica,* found only few organisms and these only for a short time in the rabbit. Geigy and Aeschlimann (305) recorded rabbits as not sensitive to *B. duttonii.* Greiner (324) succeeded in infecting young rabbits with *B. hispanica.* Baltazard *et al.* (61) were able to produce fatal infection in newborn rabbits, principally after animal passage.

Guinea pigs have developed into a favorite tool for differentiating borreliae. Greiner (324) found them refractory to *B. recurrentis.* Wolman and Wolman (736) observed, however, that guinea pigs could be infected with the Ethiopian strain of *B. recurrentis.*

Baltazard (46) pointed out that these rodents are only exceptionally susceptible to *B. recurrentis.* Coghill and Gambles (186) found that *B. recurrentis* causes only latent infection in guinea pigs, that *B. hispanica* always produces patent infection, and that these animals are refractory to South American borreliae. Kervran (409) observed elevated temperature in guinea pigs after injecting infected blood containing *B. duttonii.* Newborn guinea pigs may be more susceptible to *B. duttonii* (304). Sergent (638) produced a disease in these animals with *B. hispanica* starting with an acute attack, then becoming chronic. Colas-Belcour and Vervent (191) made similar observations. Davis (219) found guinea pigs susceptible to all North American strains of *Borrelia.*

Baltazard *et al.* (62) suggested the use of guinea pigs in the differential diagnosis of borreliae because they are highly susceptible to *B. hispanica, B. persica,* and, principally young individuals, to North American strains but not to *B. latyschewyii,* the crocidurae subgroup, and in most instances not to *B. recurrentis.* Adults, however, were refractory also to *B. duttonii* in his experience.

Different species of monkeys and apes have been found to be susceptible to various species of borreliae. Nicolle and Blaizot (532) produced transient infections in hooded monkeys with all strains of *B. recurrentis. Macaca sp.* was particularly susceptible to the Tripoli strain of relapsing fever. LeGac (439) and Baltazard (46) also observed that *Macaca* and *Cercopithecus* monkeys could be infected with ease. A mild disease resulted. *Cynocephalus* was refractory to his *B. recurrentis* strain. *B. duttonii* may cause fatal infection in monkeys (303, 304). Rhesus monkeys have been found susceptible to North American *Borrelia* strains, also to South American borreliae (68). *M. inuus* became infected with *B. hispanica* (99, 638) but minimal pathogenicity of the crocidurae subgroup was observed in *Cynocephalus.* We have found patas *(Erythrocebus patas)* mildly susceptible to North American borreliae (268). The incubation period varies according to the mode of inoculation.

Dogs have been used by Sergent (638) in the study of *B. hispanica.* Young animals were easily infected.

Chickens were recommended for experimental purposes by Kervran (409), who transmitted *B. duttonii* to them.

Hamsters have been little used in *Borrelia* experiments. Chen and Anderson (159) found them susceptible to *B. hermsii.* We were able to transmit *B. turicatae* and *B. parkerii* to them. Splenectomized hamsters infected with *B. recurrentis* were studied by Chen *et al.* (160), who saw mild disease.

Cotton rats *(Sigmodon hispidus)* were found by Varma (701) to be more susceptible to *B. turicatae* infection than were white mice.

The possibility of using the European hedgehog *(Erinaceus europaeus)* as an experimental animal was studied by Lapierrre *et al.* (435). The hedgehog was resistant to *B. duttonii,* acquired an inapparent infection when infected with borreliae of the crocidurae subgroup, was susceptible to *B. hispanica,* and became seriously ill after infection with *B. persica.* However, the response was not always clear-cut and varied with the strains of the respective species.

Some animal experiments have been carried out by unorthodox routes of inoculation.

The infection of white rats by the transnasal route, using *B. hispanica,* was successfully accomplished by Nájera Angulo (514). Joyeaux and Sautet (389) infected rats by feeding them with brains of other rats infected with *B. duttonii.* Conjunctival and peroral infection of squirrels with *B. recurrentis* was accomplished by Chung (172). Blanc *et al.* (83) produced *Borrelia*-keratitis in the rabbit eye. *B. hispanica* caused a lesion resembling syphilitic keratitis, whereas *B. duttonii* and *B. merionesi* evoked different pathologic pictures.

Chorine and Crogue (168) quantitated *B. hispanica* in guinea pigs. The multiplication of borreliae in experimental animals was also studied by Eidmann *et al.* (252) and Baltazard *et al.* (57).

Reinfection of susceptible animals is possible after several months (533, 546).

Summaries of borreliae in laboratory animals may be presented as follows. Nicholle and Anderson (526) stated that:

1. *B. duttonii* and its relatives are virulent for mice and rats, hardly at all for guinea pigs.

2. The *B. hispanica* group is equally pathogenic for mice, rats, and guinea pigs.

3. Small-rodent borreliae can infect mice but rats and guinea pigs are not sensitive. Members of this *Borrelia* group are mildly harmful or nonpathogenic for man.

Geigy (303) summarized:

1. *B. recurrentis* causes infection in monkeys, usually after 2 to

4 days' incubation, with borrelemia lasting about 4 days. Adult mice and rats are not very susceptible, developing borrelemia with various intensity. There is no residual brain damage in the infected animals.

2. *B. duttonii* is strongly pathogenic for guinea pigs, monkeys, rats, and vervets.

3. *B. hispanica* and *B. turicatae* may cause disease in guinea pigs, but some are refractory. Monkeys, rabbits, rats, and mice can be infected while young.

4. *B. venezolensis* infects rats and mice but as a rule not rabbits and guinea pigs.

We would like to emphasize that the severe response of monkeys to *B. duttonii* and that of guinea pigs to *B. persica* and *B. hispanica* are valuable laboratory aids in differentiating tick-borne Old World borreliae.

Perhaps more extensive studies are needed on animals that harbor certain borreliae in nature or become occasionally infected with them. After standardizing the route of infection, the age of the animals used, and the infective dosage, the differentiation of *Borrelia* strains may become an easier task in the laboratory.

The Interference Phenomenon

Trautmann (689) is said to have been the first to experiment with *Trypanosoma* and *Borrelia* on the same animals in 1907. He noted that rabbit serum against *B. duttonii* immobilized but did not agglutinate *T. brucei* and *vice versa.* Daels (214) confirmed these observations. Vassiliadis and Jadin (702) found that *B. hispanica* slows down *T. rhodesiense* infections but to a lesser degree than *B. duttonii* mitigates the disease caused by *T. pecaudi.* Rubinstein and Kapusto (615) believed that a new, symbiotic "race" of *Borrelia* may develop in mice in mixed infections. Kawamura (400) reported that the injection of *B. duttonii* and *B. hispanica* simultaneously causes prolonged infection in mice but that the administration of *B. hispanica* or *B. crocidurae* together with *T. brucei* prolonged the life of the mouse from 3 or 4 days to about 22 days. Vincent (707) observed that when *T. somaliense* and *Borrelia* were injected simultaneously, the incubation period was the same as when both organisms were administered separately, namely, 3 days for the *Borrelia,* and 2 to 5 for *Try-*

panosoma. The *Trypanosoma,* however, multiplied slowly and the mice did not die in 5 to 9 days as usual after injection with *T. somaliense*. The number of typanosomes increased, and began to appear in the blood periodically. Then, *T. somaliense* started to multiply and killed the mice in 30 to 40 days. Vincent believed that the reticuloendothelial system (R.E.S.) played a significant role in these variations of suppression.

Carminati (146) experimented with *B. duttonii* and *T. brucei, T. gambiense,* and *T. equiperdum* in mice. Interference between the *Borrelia* and the *Trypanosoma* strains was observed only while numerous borreliae circulated in the blood. After their disappearance, the trypanosomiasis ran its usual course. The sera of animals treated with *B. duttonii* alone did not show anti-trypanosomal antibodies. Lapierre *et al.* (434) and Larivière *et al.* (436) extended their experimental work to *B. crocidurae;* Lapierre *et al.* (433) to several strains of *B. duttonii, B. hispanica,* and *T. brucei*. Gaillard *et al.* (286) studied also *T. cruzi*.

All investigators found variations in the interference phenomenon according to the strain employed but Gaillard *et al.* (287) felt that this phenomenon could be utilized in the differential diagnosis of borreliae. Mice should be infected with the unknown strain, and *T. brucei* injected at the height of the borrelemia. If the mice survive for a long time (2 or 3 weeks), the unknown strain may be *B. duttonii* or a member of the crocidurae subgroup. If the mice die within one week, the *Borrelia* is *B. hispanica* or *B. persica*. *B. turicatae* gives variable results.

The interference phenomenon may be due to the antigenic and biological resemblance of borreliae and trypanosomes which has been pointed out repeatedly (264, 265).

Borreliae do not interfere, however, with *Spirillum minus* and *Leptospira* infections (262, 465), malaria (640a), *Coxiella (Rickettsia) burneti* (81), or coxsackie B (447) infections. Borreliae show certain cross-reactions with treponemas and *Proteus OX* strains. This will be reviewed together with the evaluation of the importance of such responses for serologic tests in the chapter on Laboratory Diagnosis.

EPIDEMIOLOGY

Human relapsing fever, a disease carried by specific insect vectors, follows the epidemiologic pattern of arthropod-borne communicable diseases. While numerous additional factors may need to be taken into consideration, our broad outline of an ecosystem in which relapsing fever thrives is as follows.

1. The presence of a sufficient number of susceptible nonimmune persons.
2. An adequate number of an efficient, infected arthropod vector, and suitable conditions for its survival and propagation.
3. Contact of man with such carriers of borreliae.
4. The readiness of the vector to feed on man.
5. The capability of the arthropod to transmit the infectious agent to man.
6. Either the ability of the arthropod to sustain *Borrelia* by transovarian transmission in its own population, or the presence of a satisfactory number of mammals with the faculty of serving as a reservoir of borreliae.

In the foregoing chapters dealing with the history of relapsing fever and lice, *Ornithodoros,* and *Borrelia,* numerous examples have been presented which illustrate ordinary as well as unconventional relationships between man, vector, and often also animal reservoir in certain biotopes. Bionomic factors conducive to novel epidemiologic situations were discussed, for instance the propensity of some *Ornithodoros (O. moubata,* and some American species) to become domesticated, herewith introducing new ecologic elements into the picture. Upholding the basic facts that louse-borne relapsing fever is epidemic, whereas tick-borne is endemic, this chapter will deal separately with the two forms of human borreliosis. Some fundamental features have to be recounted together, however, in an endeavor to create a comprehensive image of the epidemiology of borreliosis as was done by Martini (471), Gelman (315), Geigy (303), and others.

Epidemic Relapsing Fever

The epidemiology of this disease has been related up to the time of World War II in the chapter on History. Bryceson *et al.* (127) stated that 50 million persons suffered from relapsing fever during the first half of this century, with an average mortality rate of 10%. World War II and its aftermath generated about one

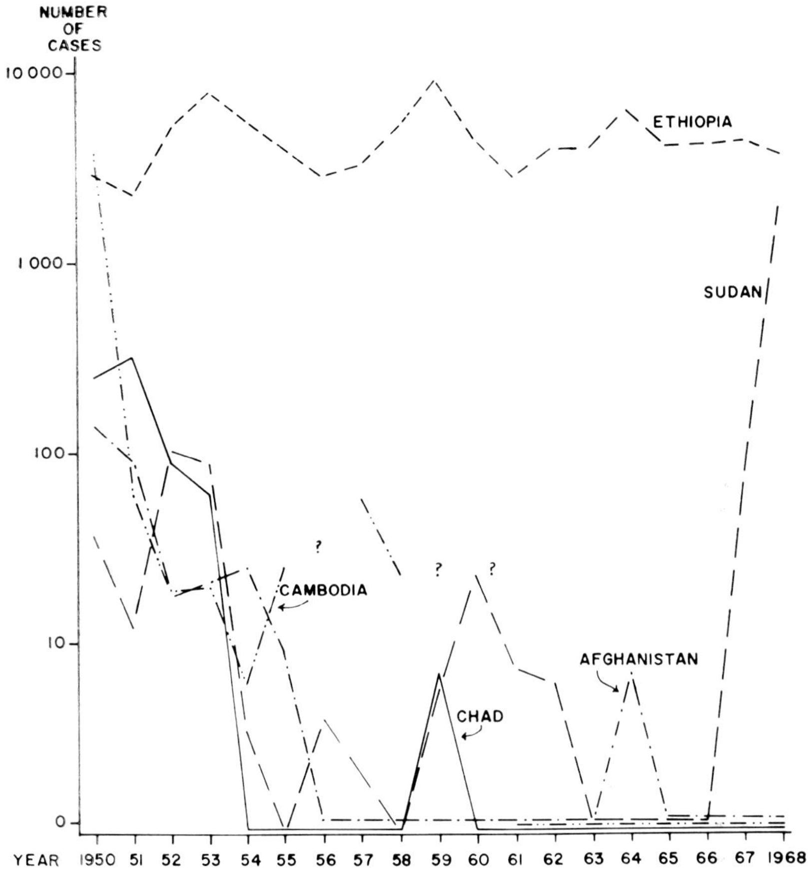

FIGURE 27. Distribution of louse-borne relapsing fever, 1950-1968, according to reports to W.H.O.

million reported infections, with about 9 million unreported cases and a 5% fatality rate, in spite of antibiotics and insecticides. These authors who studied the Abyssinian-Sudanese focus emphasized that no country is without lice. This invites attention to the ever-lasting danger of the expansion of the disease, and of the hazard of formation of new foci.

Epidemic relapsing fever has no other known reservoir than man. Admittedly, the monkey louse may transmit the causative *Borrelia,* and laboratory experiments have substantiated that non-human primates are susceptible to the disease. To the knowledge

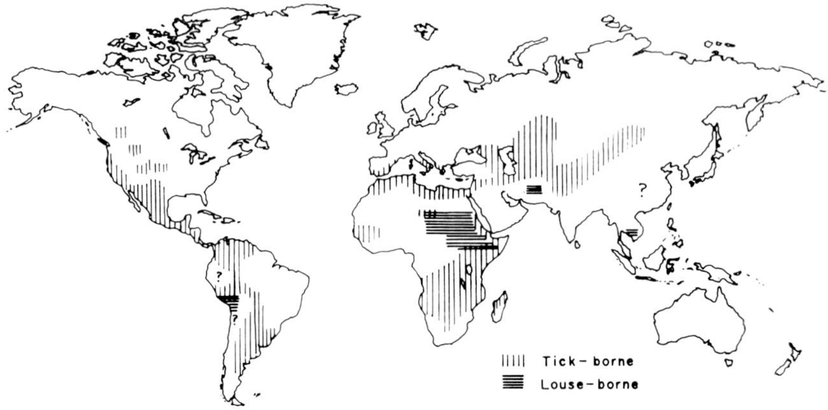

FIGURE 28. World distribution of relapsing fever, 1950-1969.

of this author, naturally infected monkey or ape populations, however, have not yet been reported. Recollecting also that the human louse does not transmit the infection to its progeny and that it has to be mutilated or killed to infect the wound resulting from its bite with celomic fluid containing borreliae, it is obvious that one louse can infect only one person, and therefore an increasing array of *P. humanus* is necessary to create an epidemic. Moreover, the infected lice must have a chance to gain access to a nonimmune person within their rather limited life span in order to transmit the infection. Such an opportunity arises when people are compelled to live in close proximity to one another.

Chung and Chang (176) enumerated conditions under which crowding of people makes it feasible for the transmission from one person to another to take place readily. Army camps, jails, poor houses, orphanages, and similar institutions, if not managed properly, may become centers of relapsing fever. Chiriboga (164) ascribed relapsing fever in Peru to poor housing, especially when living quarters were shared with animals. *P. humanus,* as a rule, however, does not feed on domestic animals. Animal husbandry so to say in the bedroom merely reduces proper hygienic conditions and diminishes living space.

The time for epidemics is the cold season (winter) when people huddle together, and heavy clothing is being worn, in which lice find a feasible microclimate. Accordingly, in hot and humid Central Africa the lightly dressed inhabitants escape lice. In Southern India, lice are found only among the very poor. Corkill (202) demonstrated that the time sequence of relapsing fever may be changed. The malady appeared in the spring in Gedaref, Sudan, being activated by kala azar infections. Baltazard *et al.* (63) observed the reappearance of the disease by the end of the winter and considered the possibility that this might have been due to a variant *Borrelia* strain. Several authors (163, 388, 645, 649) have corroborated the parallel between louse population and relapsing fever in China.

The end of the epidemic may occur when heat and humidity become high. Then the louse leaves man. At the peak of the Indian heat, during April and May, the lice begin to die (206, 207).

The seasonal occurrence of relapsing fever may be changed also by migration. Kirk (411) pointed out that migration between Egypt, Sudan, and the former French West Africa was accompanied by the introduction of infested lice. More will be given about this in the discussion of the epidemiology in Abyssinia. Chiao (163) observed also the spread of relapsing fever along highways in China, which resulted in about 5,500 cases among people associated with wayside inns and farmers living along the routes. Lanzo and Tresca (432), commenting on 2,914 cases in the former Erythrea Colony, also saw a shift from the classic winter relapsing fever season to June-September because of the time of labor migration.

People on the move, like migrant laborers, nomads, vagrants, pilgrims, sheep herders, and cattle dealers (260), acquire lice more easily than permanently settled segments of the populace, with the exception of those who live in crowded quarters with insufficient means for good hygienic practices, but including inhabitants of very cold mountainous regions who seldom change their clothing. Old clothes dealers may acquire and spread lice (154). The disease was introduced by this means from Arabia to Kenya in 1945 (296). Persons frequenting markets in which infested clothing is offered for sale, or those who come in contact with louse-carrying animal dealers moving about, also may become infected (260).

On the other hand, nonimmune immigrants entering infected areas, as in Abyssinia, principally seasonal laborers and job-seekers who live under poor conditions, may acquire *Borrelia*-infested lice, and the disease.

Age and sex susceptibility seems to exist only as far as the opportunity of acquiring *Borrelia*-bearing lice and the mode of crushing them are concerned. It has been mentioned before that in China and South America lice are often popped between the teeth. Some authors believed that borreliae can enter the body only through abrasions (462), others have cited examples of infection through intact mucosae, such as Legge (440) and L'Abbate and Mannino (429) who reported borreliosis developing after instillation of infected blood into the conjunctivae. The presently prevailing belief is that borreliae may enter the human body through uninjured mucosae, including that of the gastrointestinal tract (135) (see also chapter on Portal of Entry). The popping of lice between the teeth may lead to an increased number of relapsing fever infections, principally among adults. The age and sex distribution of migrants favors males as the victims of relapsing fever. Chung and Chang (176) found the ratio of males to females 6 to 1 in China, Bryceson *et al.* (127) 3 to 1 in Abyssinia. The latter authors observed the disease principally among young males, as did Robertson (606) in China.

During wars and other disasters, such as earthquakes, famines, fires, and floods, people are often compelled to flee in masses, and to live in congested quarters. Water is usually scarce, clothing is not properly washed, and conditions become favorable for the multiplication of lice. Then relapsing fever epidemics break out.

The great epidemic of World War II is believed to have started in Fezzan in Southern Tripolitania in 1943, according to Gaud and Morgan (298), where the first cases of the 1912 epidemic were also observed. Nomads of the Megarha tribe were supposed to have harbored the infection. Sparrow (664) pointed out, however, that the disease may have been imported from Abyssinia which was at that time, as was Tripoli, under Italian rule. As a matter of fact, the first patient with relapsing fever in neighboring Tunisia was an Italian prisoner of war (323). The epidemic swept through North Africa in 1943-1945, Egypt in 1945-1946, Ethiopia, Sudan, and Nigeria in 1947-1948, Kenya in 1945, then the Near and Far East (297, 298, 303, 500).

During this epidemic Stuart (670) observed that the disease

was at first mild in Tunisia, Algeria, and Morocco, but later became severe with a 10 to 12% mortality. Gaud and Morgan (298) reported a 50% morbidity rate in 1942-1944. This was probably due to lack of herd immunity because relapsing fever was absent from that area for 25 years. Bryceson *et al.* (127), commenting on the 20-year periodicity of relapsing fever in Africa, remarked that this may be the time needed for a nonimmune population to grow up, or it may be caused by military activities recurring after two decades — in 1903, 1923, 1943.

The actual number of cases in North Africa is unknown. Among those recorded by Graeves *et al.* (323), the mortality varied between 1 and 46% in Tunisia, according to the locality. The disease subsided in Tunisia after 2 years, then invaded neighboring countries. Algeria had a 5% morbidity. To the West, Nigeria reported mild cases imported from Morocco to Dakar and Tiaroye Camp.

Spanish Morocco was infected from the former French Morocco. Between March-July 1945, 168 cases were reported. To the East, Egypt was plagued simultaneously by louse-borne typhus and a relapsing fever epidemic. Halwani (333) and Kamal *et al.* (395) stated that about 100,000 persons became ill. Gaud and Morgan (298) described the spread of the disease to Iran, Jordan, Syria, Aden, and Palestine, where only scattered instances were observed, while Iran and Kenya experienced true epidemics. There were 200 cases in Haifa (332). The disease in Kenya was studied by Heisch (340). The aftermaths of the introduction of relapsing fever from Seihut, South Arabia, to Mombasa, Kenya, by several dhows carrying patients who imported the disease, has been demonstrated by the observation of isolated cases by Ombati and Ojiambo (553). Saglan (621) commented upon the mild outbreak in Turkey. The disease reached true epidemic proportions, however, in Abadan, Iran, in November 1945 to June 1946, with 1,087 cases, commencing after an unusual cold spell. This was the first extensive louse-borne relapsing fever epidemic recorded in Iran. Head lice were found on 88% of the patients, and *B. recurrentis* was isolated from some of these ectoparasites. It is not certain that the small outbreak in Northeast Bengal, with 9 laborers becoming ill, was related to the large World War II epidemic (152).

In Europe, Yugoslavia suffered both from louse-borne typhus

and relapsing fever. Serstnev (644) believed that residual endemic foci may still exist in that country.

Romania had about 4,000 cases according to Gaud *et al.* (297) but Zaharia (744) saw 58 cases daily in 1945 and 1946 in a single hospital. Exact statistics are not available from Poland. Lipinski (453) reported a milder course of the disease than during World War I, with a 0.25% case fatality rate. He ascribed this to prompt treatment with arsenicals.

The epidemic reached Hungary from Rumania in 1945 (570). Eighty to 85% of the cases occurred among gypsies who had been relocated in settlements at that time; one-half of all the ill were in the age group between 10 and 29 years. The case fatality rate was 3.7%.

No data are available from the U.S.S.R. It is possible that the *Febris neuralgica periodica,* misnamed also 5-day fever (101), was actually relapsing fever. Böger (88) observed and correctly diagnosed the disease in German troops in the Southern U.S.S.R.

The World War II epidemic also reached Portugal where isolated cases were seen (578) and Spain where it was called "vagabond fever". Sabalette *et al.* (620) studied 30 cases in Sevilla, and Forteza Bover *et al.* (276) 5 in Valencia. This was the first recorded invasion of Spain by louse-borne relapsing fever.

War-connected relapsing fever may be louse-borne, as it was in Korea among the population infested with DDT-resistant lice (17), but it may be tick-borne as in Israel (420) or in India (165) when troops enter caves and tick-infested shelters.

After the World War II epidemic subsided, Afghanistan reported 138 cases in 1958 and a few in 1964. Afghanistan is mountainous, dry, and cold. Such areas are favorable for relapsing fever. Unfortunately, few (or no) data are available from the Pamir, the Himalayas, and from many of the South American highlands. At the other extreme lies hot and wet Cambodia with 4,216 reports in 1950. The number of cases decreased to 6 in 1954, and a few were reported in 1957 and 1958. Although no accounts are available from Mainland China and North Viet Nam, it is possible that louse-borne borreliae are being imported from those countries to Cambodia. On the other hand, isolated foci in Cambodia may be residua of the epidemics during the first part of this century, perhaps brought in by migrant tribes or remaining active in isolated spots.

According to the reports reaching the World Health Organization (20), Abyssinia had 2,860 cases in 1950. The number of annually reported instances increased to 7,499 in 1953 and 8,760 in 1959, with a low of 2,760 in 1961. The number increased to 5,971 in 1964 and came to 3,729 in 1968. All provinces are infected at present (1969-1970) and the number of reported cases has not been below 2,760 in any year between 1950 and 1968.

The Sudan had less than 100 cases per year until 1953, then very few until 1967 when 70 instances were reported, and 1,948 in 1968. This has to be considered a veritable epidemic. All five provinces of the Sudan are now infected.

Developments in the Chad followed the opposite path. A few hundred cases were reported in 1950 and 1951, less than 100 in 1952 and 1953, very few in 1959, then none. Fig. 27 shows the fluctuations in the number of cases reported to the World Health Organization on a logarithmic scale. It has to be remembered that only louse-borne but not tick-borne cases are reportable according to the International Sanitary Regulations now in force (379).

The great number of cases in Ethiopia and the Sudan deserve further attention.

Bryceson *et al.* (127) pointed out that the Abyssinian highlands are cold, principally during the local winter (June-September), where agent, vector, and susceptible host coincide. There are numerous susceptible seasonal laborers and job-seekers coming to Addis Ababa and its environs. Historically, the war between the Mahdists and Christians on the Ethiopian Plateau in the 1880's is of interest. Few of the defeated Mahdists moved away but there was an exodus for religious reasons to Chad in 1894. Chad is on the pilgrimage path from West Africa to Mecca, as well as on the trade route from North Africa. When the followers of Rabih Zubair were defeated in 1900, they moved probably along the latter trail to Fezzan, Algeria, and Tunisia (127). According to these authors relapsing fever was first diagnosed in the Adua and Axum outbreaks in 1918. Italian physicians in Ethiopia and British troops faced the disease during the war (646). Ethiopian outbreaks have been recorded by several writers (156, 607, 608, 661, 664, 736), as well as the export of the disease to Kenya (296) and its movement from and to the Sudan (411). Sparrow (664) and Bryceson *et al.* (127) consider Ethiopia a highly important epidemic focus, with about 1,000 cases and 5% mortality per year in Addis Ababa. Relapsing fever in Ethiopia is at home also in the South-West Highlands especially among seasonal coffee bean pickers, along the railroad from the Red Sea Coast, and in the lowlands of Jijiga, where the tick-borne form is also present.

Whereas *B. hispanica,* an Eastasian tick, followed the route of the Moslem Conquest to the West, *B. recurrentis,* probably of African origin, spread by war and migration to all parts of the world except Australia, New Zealand, and Polynesia. Tick-borne borreliae have become louse-adapted in the laboratory but have not mutated into the epidemic strain. Lice do not transmit borreliae to their progeny by the transovarian (hereditary) route, which is contrary to most *Borrelia*-bearing ticks. Each vector-louse has to be infested individually, and less than 20% of the lice fed on patients are able to transmit the disease. The presence of infected man or some other, hitherto unknown reservoir appears to be a *condicio sine qua non* for the maintenance of relapsing fever caused by the epidemic strain, *B. recurrentis,* or else tick-borne borreliae mutate into a louse-borne type by a hitherto undiscovered mechanism. The continuity of louse-borne relapsing fever, demonstrated by Bryceson *et al.* (127), certainly speaks in favor of contiguous and continuous man-to-man transmission, while *O. moubata* and lice feeding on the same persons in Africa yet offer food for thought and consideration along another course.

Endemic Relapsing Fever

Endemic relapsing fever is tick-borne. Its ecology coincides with that of *Ornithodoros* species carrying human pathogenic borreliae. The occurrence of this type of relapsing fever also depends on the frequency of contact between man and arthropod. Man and *Ornithodoros* meet according to the life habits of the species involved. *O. moubata,* dwelling in huts inhabited by man, will have a greater and more frequent opportunity to feed on him and transfer borreliae to man than will *O. parkeri,* which avoids human abodes. Man may, however, invade the habitats of the tick as a temporary visitor (hunter, vacationer, soldier, and so forth), or as a permanent resident when new lands are opened for cultivation and new roads are built.

Tick-borne relapsing fever is usually at home within the 24°C summer isotherm (471). *Ornithodoros* do not live in the monsoon and rain forests. They occur in semi-desert areas, but man seldom goes there. In colder climates these arthropods are active only during the warm season, but all year around in the tropics. The feeding time of the nymphs and adult ticks usually coincides with the period when relapsing fever is most frequent. In the Kashmir, however, ticks breed during the winter, but relapsing fever is most frequent in the summer (394) when man more often invades the habitats of ticks.

Lice have to be crushed to transfer *Borrelia.* They die as a result of such an injury and thus can infect only one person. However, ticks do not have to be damaged to transfer the borreliae they carry. A single *Ornithodoros* may infect a different person or animal at each feeding. Adult ticks usually transfer borreliae through their coxal fluid, which is excreted during or after feeding. Some ticks, especially young specimens and developmental forms, may transmit borreliae with their bite. Since ticks do not move far from their burrows, they infect only man and animals that enter their limited area. Some *Ornithodoros,* as *O. moubata,* seldom move farther than about 20 meters under their own power. However, they can be carried by man or animals to new locations and may originate new endemic foci but not epidemics.

At present, the best known foci of tick-borne relapsing fever are in Northwest and West Iran (591), in the desert-steppe regions of Central Asia (564), in Azerbeidjan principally on the Aspheron Peninsula (39, 585), in Soviet Georgia (746), Southwest Turkestan (586), Turkmenia (566), Kazakhstan (651), Uzbekistan (657), along the Southwest Littoral of the Mediterranean (686), in the Arab countries (36), Israel (253), Kenya, Tanzania, and Uganda (303), South Africa (556), the Kashmir (600), in the Western part of the United States (69, 740), especially in Oklahoma (274), Kansas (183), Texas (195, 722), Oregon (218,

283, 356), and California (70, 652).* Only scattered cases have been reported in the United States with the exception of an incident involving a small scout troop which visited a cave infested with *O. turicata* in Kansas (U.S. Communicable Diseases Center report). Several other occurrences of tick-borne relapsing fever were discussed in the chapter on *Ornithodoros* and the borreliae carried by them.

Reports from South America are meager. Marinkelle and Grose 474) isolated an unidentified *Borrelia* species from a bat *(Natalus tumidirostris)* in the large Maceregue cave near San Gil, in Colombia. This indicates that borreliosis is still present in that country. Vigors Earle (705) reported tick-borne relapsing fever in Ecuador, Colombia, and Venezuela.

An interesting summary of the relationship of the types of human habitations to the tick population was published by Walton (715). In regions where ticks are not infested in large numbers, the infection may be smoldering. An example is Madagascar, where *B. duttonii* is maintained by transovarian passage in relatively few individual *O. moubata* (189, 517). In Panama, the proportion of *Borrelia*-infested ticks may not have changed recently, but since canvas cots are replacing the old board or bamboo beds the ticks have been deprived of their hiding places, which has resulted in a lower infection rate in man (182).

As stated, soldiers, hunters, laborers, and tourists entering tick-infested areas are frequent victims of relapsing fever (137, 182). Local inhabitants of endemic areas may have acquired a certain degree of immunity during childhood (73). Therefore, it is principally the newcomer who becomes ill in such regions (705). This was the case in Cyprus during World War II where tick-borne *Borrelia* infestations were discovered also in local miners (291, 738). Tick-borne relapsing fever appeared in 41 soldiers entering native huts in Transvaal (492), in troops and travelers moving along tick-infested roads in Madagascar (189, 430), in the caravanserais of Iran (245, 739), and in the mountains of California where hunters and vacationers had used abandoned huts often infested with ticks (729). An episode of tick-borne relapsing fever

*Thompson *et al.* (J.A.M.A., *210*:1045, 1969) recently called attention to tick-borne relapsing fever also in the State of Washington.

in children who followed a porcupine into a cave was described in Palestine (6). Bates *et al.* (68) studied 6 cases in boys who went hunting in the Arriján area of Panama, were badly bitten by ticks, and developed relapsing fever. Konitzer (419) reported the occurrence of the disease in Arabs sleeping in a cave. Severe relapsing fever developed in soldiers visiting caves near Damascus (625). Cooper (201) found infected soldiers who had acquired the disease in caves, old dugouts, tank traps, and trenches infested with rodents in Tobruk. An identical situation developed in Cyprus (291, 738). Ashbel (29) compared the strains isolated from soldiers in Tobruk and Palestine, and found some differences. But soldiers off duty also may acquire tick-borne relapsing fever, such as one who chased a porcupine into a cave near Jerusalem (253).

Many infested ticks live in the desert areas of Africa (471), in the less inhabited regions of Central Asia (33, 398, 571), and in the Caspian area (39, 475, 746). Their contacts with man are few, and therefore the human infection rate is low. Sometimes the tick vector is associated with domestic animals, as with sheep in the Kashmir (394), and create a hazard to their tenders; or with fowl kept in living huts, as in East Africa (432). The huts in East Africa abound with tick vectors of *Borrelia* (338, 340).

It is said that indigenous people from East Africa carry *O. moubata* with them for good luck. This tick becomes easily domesticated. The relapsing fever in the Witwatersrand gold mines (742), and among other migrant Africans in South Africa (19), is a disease imported by man. Geigy (303) attempted to acquire "good-luck" ticks from these people for investigating the borreliae in them but did not succeed. *O. moubata* not dwelling with man is irregularly distributed in Africa but its ecology in the wild is the same as that of the warthog (303, 711). Geigy found it in the hair of warthogs which are hunted, and agrees with Walton (711) that the original habitat of *O. moubata,* the vector of *B. duttonii,* was probably with those animals but then the arthropod was transferred to huts by man carrying warthog pelts or carcasses.

Other *Ornithodoros* (principally *O. tholozani)* move with caravans, on sheep, camels, and other animals driven from one place to another, and may make their homes in used or abandoned stopover places along the caravan route. Considering that *O. tholozani* may live for more than 20 years and transmit the infection after 10 years (108, 568), the survival of *B. persica,* the organism carried by it, appears to be rather well insured. One frequently encounters quite dried-out and apparently lifeless *O. moubata* and *O. tholozani* which avidly feed and return to normal at the first occasion when blood becomes available.

The parasite-vector-host relationships in relapsing fever may be delicately balanced, or the association may be based on less specific factors. There is no firm indication to date that the human louse feeds on mammals other than man outside the laboratory. Numerous *Borrelia*-bearing *Ornithodoros* bite several species of animals, whereas others display more selective food habits. *Ornithodoros* may use the burrows, caves, and other types of shelters of animals with or without feeding on them. The species of rodent or cold-blooded animal inhabitants of such hiding places may change, but the tick may remain in the shelter because it often selects a particular habitat rather for the microclimate (temperature, moisture, etc.) than because of the animals living in it. If a tick infested with borreliae feeds on an animal, it does not necessarily infect the animal, and the mammalian host of the tick does not always become a reservoir of *Borrelia.*

Another factor that limits the role of mammals in the cycle of borreliosis is their reaction to the bite of the tick. Some ticks produce local analgesia. The bite of others is so painful that the animal will become aware of the tick and try to get rid of it. Several species of ticks feed for a long time, others for only 20 to 60 minutes. *Ornithodoros* that successfully transmit borreliae to man belong to the latter category. Those that are night-feeders and attack man in his sleep are the most effective propagators of borreliae. Baltazard *et al.* (56) correlated the response of younger and older animals to tick bite and found that young animals, which are less able to rid themselves of ticks and which have a higher mortality rate when infected with *Borrelia,* become the prime victims of borreliosis when ticks are hatching and seek food. A more stable state develops when only mature animals are present in the burrows and dugouts.

The vector-host relationship becomes further involved when

Ornithodoros seeks to share the shelters of domestic animals or feed on them. A broad field for cooperative studies in a hitherto little investigated area can be entered here.

PATHOLOGY

In terms of the present functional or "dynamic" concept of pathology, borreliosis is a disease characterized by cyclic responses to a cyclic agent. The problem is why these changes take place in man. Epidemics are not always feasible for detailed studies because of the large number of patients to be treated, the habitually crowded and undermanned facilities in louse-infested areas as well as in sparsely inhabited regions where *Ornithodoros* thrives, and the lack of interest in this illness in advanced countries where the disease is rare, often merely meriting a case report in a local medical journal. Well-equipped laboratories, therefore, have resorted principally to animal experimentation in the past. The animal models used have been mostly rodents, which are phylogenetically remote from man, and do not permit drawing conclusions valid

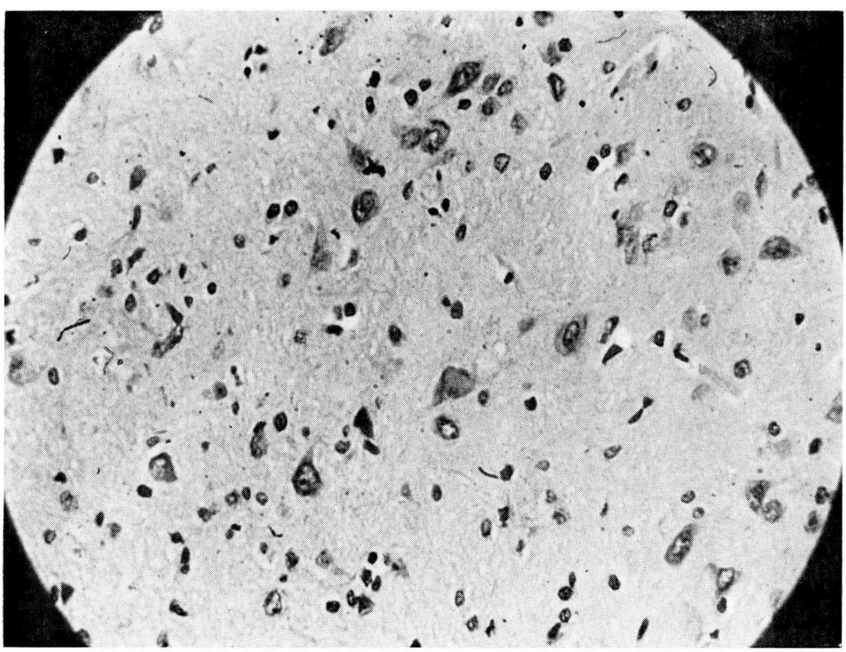

FIGURE 29. Gliosis and neuron cell damage in relapsing fever.

for human beings in all aspects. Nevertheless much of our present-day knowledge of borreliosis is derived from rodent experiments, which will be summarized first.

Predisposition to borreliosis has not been studied to a great extent. One of the most important results of such investigations is that of Guggenheim *et al.* (328, 329) who demonstrated that protein and thiamine-deficient diet predisposes rats to severe *B. persica* infection. This may have been due also to the concomitant caloric deficiency.

In young rats infected with *B. merionesi,* the borreliae were found only inside veins, terminal arteries, capillaries, and sinusoids including those of the bone marrow but no inflammatory changes were noted and no phagocytosis. Small necrotic areas in different organs were due to obstruction of the circulation by blood coagula (446). In other infections, in Central Asia, borreliae were always fewer in the blood than in the spleen of the rodents. Neither phagocytosis, nor disintegrating borreliae could be detected by Aravantinos (22). Kritschewski and Singinshima (422) considered phagocytosis an accidental phenomenon in which fixed phagocytes do not play a role, and only dead organisms are attacked by phagocytes.

The reticuloendothelial system (R.E.S.) has been considered important in borreliosis because when it is blocked in otherwise resistant animals, these may become susceptible to borreliae (126, 736). Borreliae are destroyed in the body by antibodies, not by phagocytes (393). The anatomy of the brain with respect to the blood supply apparently is the reason that borreliae are less exposed to antibodies in the central nervous system (C.N.S.) than they are in the blood stream. It is not known, however, why the "neurotropism" of some borreliae differs from that of others.

Splenectomized animals often but not always had more borreliae in their circulation than surgically unaltered rodents. Pirot and Bourgain (581) but not Baltazard (46, 50) found splenectomy more effective in producing serious *Borrelia* disease. In *B. duttonii* infections there seemed to be some relationship between the reticulocyte response, the blood loss, the development of anemia, and the number of borreliae injected, in the trials conducted by Robertson (605). *B. persica* caused severe bleeding, including hemoperitoneum (119). Kemp *et al.* (404) observed splenic enlargement and a decrease of younger cells in the perifocal zones, only small lymphocytes in the germinal centers, some of these with pyknotic nuclei, and dilated sinuses tightly packed with red blood cells, without hemolysis and phagocytosis of the red blood cells in the splenic sinuses.

The so-called *B. novyi* served in the experiments of Martínez Báez and Villasana (470). They found the capillaries of the pia mater, cerebrum, and cerebellum, as well as the choroid plexus, congested. There was a microglial response in the cerebral cortex, and the cornu ammonis. No changes were apparent in the neurons. Lymphocytic infiltration of the pia with later absorption of small hemorrhages was observed. Garnham *et al.* (296), however, saw degeneration of the ganglion cells without meningovascular inflammation, in Kenya.

Rats infected with *B. recurrentis* produced large amounts of lactic acid, followed by a blood carbon dioxide shift, hypoglycemia, and glycogen depletion (385).

It is interesting to note that Horrenberger (372) found *B. hispanica* also in the saliva of infected guinea pigs.

Kemp *et al.* (404) believed that the periodicity of the disease in man is due rather to a refractory period of the borreliae than to antibody activity. In our concept, this statement has to be amplified and modified in view of recent clinical and experimental evidence. For instance, the development of antibodies against subsequent phase variants which begins shortly before the crisis (136) and steadily increases during subsequent attacks (265, 268, 303), together with the slow ascent of the levels of avid antibody leading to firm antibody-antigen complexes in primates, may explain the dilatory evolution of immunity. The reluctance of borreliae to enter tissues and remain within the arteriovenous and capillary bed and interstitial spaces as well as the lack of participation of a considerable proportion of the R.E.S. may account for the slow process of antibody formation *via* the RNA-polysomal route.* The assumptions of Russell (618), Belezki and Umanskaya (72), and Bryceson *et al.* (127) that antibodies immobilize and begin to

*Our recent experiments in patas monkeys (Exptl. Molec. Path., *12:255*, 1970) demonstrated the role of tRNA-ribosomal participation in this process.

lyse borreliae, after which phagocytosis may take place, with R.E.S. playing the role of a filter, was borne out by Anderson and Zimmerman (17) and others. Schofield *et al.* (629) pointed out the role of leukocytes during the crisis which ends the attacks. The theory of such a role is based on immunoadherence (3) and leukotaxis which may unmask new determinants according to Bryceson *et al.* (127), particularly the release of endogenous pyrogen from these elements. Parry *et al.* (562) demonstrated also that the white blood cells, which abruptly decrease in number before the crisis and return to normal after the borreliae disappear from the circulation, often are vacuolated and show loss of granules. Schofield *et al.* (629) felt that this is rather sequestration than loss of a large number of cells because the serum muramidase (lysozyme) does not increase.

Russell (617, 618) had already observed as early as 1930 that macrophages do not phagocytize borreliae but that pinocytosis (engulfing of dead fragments) takes place in them. Hindle (364) felt, however, that R.E.S. plays a greater role in the destruction of borreliae and that these cells actively respond to borreliae. Borreliae seem to break up in the spleen (618) but fixed phages do not engulf them there (404). Anderson and Zimmerman (17) believed that the process in the spleen is of considerable importance for disposing of borreliae. It is not known how borreliae are actually killed (631), principally since polymorphonuclear cells have been said to phagocytize only dead borreliae (669). We join those who believe that the organisms appear to be destroyed by antibodies rather than by phagocytosis (393, 422, 688).

Borreliae retreat to the central nervous system, the spleen, the liver, and the bone marrow after the primary attack and after each relapse (68, 133, 235, 591, 620, 640, 731, 732). As a result of infection with *Borrelia,* there are antibodies present against that organism, but the levels of antibodies in the cerebrospinal fluid are significantly lower than in the blood (719). It is known, however, that borreliae penetrate the blood-cerebrospinal barrier (281).

The literature on white blood cells is richly documented. Karwacki and Krakowska (397), and Bryceson *et al.* (127) found an increased white blood cell count in relapsing fever, with an abrupt fall just before the borreliae disappear from the blood, then a return to normal. Others (482, 503) emphasized a shift to the left, with monocytosis and eosinopenia. In *B. duttonii* infections, low eosinophil counts seem to be the rule (437). The same observation was made in louse-borne relapsing fever (387, 127). Sulday (672), in Madagascar, saw an increase in polymorphonuclear neutrophiles during the attack. Lymphocytes also increased while eosinophils decreased in number. Monocyte counts reached their lowest point just before the febrile episode, and their maximum at the beginning of the interim. Karwacki and Krakowska (397) found an increase in lymphocyte counts in the crisis; when this did not occur, a relapse followed. Other authors (175, 176, 590) made similar observations. Browse (114) did not find marked changes in the blood picture in his patients in Qetta.

Another feature of relapsing fever is the involvement of the blood circulation. Capillaries impacted with red blood cells, or a hemolytic tendency (17) due to lack of one or two coagulation factors (127), may cause petechiae or more serious profuse bleeding, and ischemic, then necrotic foci in any organ. This may result in central nervous system, lung, gastrointestinal, and other disturbances. Considering further hematologic changes, the hemoglobin is usually low (404, 503); Más de Ayala (476) found it seldom unchanged. Bryceson *et al.* (127) pointed out that in high altitudes such as in Addis Ababa the ratio of hemoglobin to the red cell count may differ from that at lower altitudes. Polychromasia and poikilocytosis (672); progressive anemia of the hypochromic and normocytic type (388) in China; at times also hemolytic anemia (299) has been observed in Israel. Robinson (607) saw prothrombin deficit. This was measured by Bryceson *et al.* (127) in terms of a prolonged prothrombin time. These authors also recorded lowered fibrinogen levels and decreased clotting ability of the blood. The bleeding time was unchanged. Few alterations in the serum chemistry were noted by Maruashvilli (475) in the Caucasus in mild tick-borne infections.

Cimmino (181) reported an increased blood sedimentation rate (BSR) both during attacks and remissions in Erithrea. Increased BSR was also registered in Somaliland (156) and in Israel (253). The platelet count was nearly always low in Abyssinia and in Israel. Extensive hemorrhages may occur also in borreliosis in South

America (573). These and the petechial rash will be discussed under Clinical Symptoms.

The postmortem changes are not specific (71). Russell (617) described focal necrosis in the spleen. El Ramly (255) saw infarcts, mostly in males, during the first attack of louse-borne relapsing fever, which often become septic. Perisplenitis, in addition to miliary necrosis, has been reported (607), as well as miliary lesions, congestion, and infiltration around the follicles, sometimes with tangled masses of borreliae in the germinal centers, at times marginal leukocytic infiltrations accompanied by mononuclears and fibrin (404).

A further feature of relapsing fever is hepatitis which was emphasized by Bryceson *et al.* (127). Mayer (482) believed that borreliae stay in the liver and are slowly released during the attacks. The liver is sometimes enlarged and the lobules less distinct than normally. Kemp *et al.* (404) reported parenchymatous degeneration with enlarged cells harboring pyknotic nuclei. The sinuses appeared narrow but congested, the endothelial cells prominent. The number of Kupffer cells may be increased. Judge and Perine (391) related similar findings. The disturbances in the liver functions are reflected in increased serum bilirubin, alkaline phosphatase, and the transaminases S.G.O.T. and S.G.P.T. values. These features were systematically studied by Bryceson *et al.* (127); and reported also by Ombati and Oijambo (553); and Eisenberg *et al.* (253). The urine may be dark (127), frequently with bile pigments (476). Urobilin and urobilinogen were found in Cyprus (242) and in other localities where liver involvement was recorded. Liver damage apparently is a frequent finding in severe cases.

There may be renal changes, principally in the tubules. The kidney may be congested and enlarged. The cells of the convoluted tubules are often swollen, and irregular. Hyaline casts may be seen in the urine. The interstitial tissue shows cellular infiltration, but the Bowman capsules are seldom involved. Bryceson *et al.* (127) often found proteinuria with leukocytes and also erythrocytes in the urine. Microscopic hematuria is said to be more common in tick than in louse-borne relapsing fever. Exceptions to this man-made rule were registered by Chang (154), but renal infarcts are always a possibility (253). Proteinuria was noted (74) practically in all instances early in the disease; Pifano (573) observed it during the later course of the disease. Urinary findings resembling those of nephrosis have been recorded (176, 298, 469).

There is fluid loss (464) due to sweating and fast breathing. Blood urea nitrogen is increased. Plasma Na and K are increased but not constantly; Cl is often low in borreliosis in Abyssinia according to Bryceson *et al.* (127). These authors also noted an increase in gamma globulin, possibly changes in beta globulin, and a decrease of alpha globulins and albumin in some sera.

The "neurotropism" of borreliae has been a constantly recurring puzzle. It may be strain-specific because reports on species-specificity list too many exceptions. The infection of the C.N.S. may be latent (133). Garnham *et al.* (296) found, in louse-borne relapsing fever of Kenya, degeneration of the ganglion cells of the cerebellum without meningovascular changes but stated that glia cell reactions may be extensive. *B. recurrentis* may remain in the C.S.F. for 65 to 69 days (582, 583). Borreliae were found in the C.S.F., in the brain, as well as in brain tumors, in East Africa (590). Increased globulin was observed in the C.S.F. (175). Lodewyckx (454) noted lymphocytosis in the spinal fluid principally in *B. duttonii* infections. The clinical picture appears to be dominated by the consequences of the hemodynamic changes in the C.N.S., their localization, and extent.

The heart may show endocarditis (607). Other authors (17, 391) have emphasized myocardial changes seen at autopsy. Hemorrhages of various size may be found in practically every organ.

Borreliae in the skin and the histology of the hemorrhages were studied by Taft and Pike (674) who found the organisms in the skin also between attacks, and by Judge and Perine (391) who investigated biopsy specimens.

Abortion is very frequent. About 92% of pregnant women lose their children when they contract relapsing fever (552).

It is expected that the variations of the borreliae, their particular predilection for certain localizations, the uncommon immunologic responses, together with the hemodynamic changes analyzed by Parry *et al.* (562) may assist in understanding the motley and protean clinical course of relapsing fever.

CLINICAL PICTURE

Attempts have been made to demonstrate a common denominator or to establish differential diagnostic criteria between louse-borne and tick-borne relapsing fever. Since we are confronted with one or more agents of varied pathogenicity and organotropy, with changes in the course of the illness according to epidemics and localities as well as with sick people but not diseases *per se,* this task is rather difficult if not impossible.

Clinical Course

The clinical course of relapsing fever has been described by several authors, such as Calwell (139), Selwyn-Clarke *et al.* (636), Robertson (606), Robinson (608), Davidson (215), Banwell and Kibukamusoka (67), Whitmore (731, 732), Bryceson *et al.* (127), and others to whom frequent reference will be made in this chapter.

Generally speaking, the course of human relapsing fever consists of an incubation period, the first attack, and, at intervals, of relapses. The typical "relapse course" is not always followed. There may be an irregular temperature curve (149, 345) or only one febrile attack (657). The severity of the disease often depends on circumstances which deserve further discussion even though the currently used classification (443) into severe, mild, ambulant, latent, and atypical forms, is of considerable use for recording.

Severity of the Disease

Tick-borne relapsing fever is usually more severe and more prolonged than the louse-borne type (149). There is an amazing variability, however, from outbreak to outbreak, as well as from one area to another. Individual susceptibility and residual immunity also may be important. While, for instance, in North and in East Africa *Borrelia* infections are severe in Europeans and mild in the local population (467, 642), in West Africa relapsing fever is equally severe in both Europeans and Africans. Variations in the severity of the disease according to geography are also interesting. Louse-borne relapsing fever was very severe in 1912 in Indochina (495) and in Gurkha laborers in Darjeeling (392), but it was very mild in Turkey and Egypt (139). Tick-borne infections have been described as severe in Central Africa (685) and in Syria and Lebanon (624), mild in Israel (420) and West Pakistan (114), very mild in the Asian U.S.S.R. (655), but they show a wide variety of intensity in the Americas (443, 464). The severity of the disease seems to decline with the duration of the epidemic type caused by *B. recurrentis.*

B. hispanica infections are usually mild, as are those due to the crocidurae subgroup. This differs from the frequently severe *B. persica* infections. In the Americas, *B. hermsii* has been causing severe illness, *B. turicatae* usually mild disease, and *B. venezolensis* sickness of variable intensity.

Symptoms of relapsing fever, as shown above, vary with the immunity of the host, the strain of *Borrelia* that is involved, the phase of the epidemic, and a number of other less known or unknown factors. There are indications also that relapsing fever may exist with few or no clinical manifestations, particularly in endemic areas.

It is questionable from the clinical point of view if the "one day fever" often caused by *B. latyschewii* should be called relapsing fever *sensu stricto.*

Incubation Period

The incubation period was established partly by studying patients with general paresis who had been infected with *Borrelia* for therapeutic purposes, partly by epidemiologic observations, and, to a lesser extent, by experiments on volunteers.

In louse-borne relapsing fever the incubation time is 2 to 15 days, usually 5 to 8 days (176, 467, 503, 620). In Abyssinia, the incubation time is 4 to 14 days (127). Exceptions have been reported. One of these was that of two boys from Romania who became ill in Liverpool after having left their country 17 days previously, and were free from lice (542). Infection through the conjunctiva has produced disease in 8 days (429).

The incubation period of tick-borne relapsing fever in Asia and Africa could be established in several instances by determining the time that had elapsed since the individual visited a cave, a hut, or some other area where the tick vectors dwell. Geigy (303) observed it for 2 to 10 days in *O. moubata* infections. The incubation period in military operations in Tobruk (201) and in Cyprus (739) was approximately 9 days. In Palestine and Israel (6, 253) it was 5 to 9 days, usually 7 to 8; in Tashkent (398) 6 to 14 days; in the Caucasus (475) 6 to 10 days; and in Mozambique (469) it was 5 to 14 days. *B. graingeri* caused clinical symptoms after 10 days (345). A very short incubation period was observed in North Africa (476), 2 to 4 days, while after infections with organisms of the crocidurae group (53), and from South Africa, periods of 4 to 12 days have been reported (469, 557).

Baltazard *et al.* (63) stated that the incubation period may depend on the number of borreliae that have penetrated into the body.

Observations of the incubation period made by feeding infected ticks on human volunteers had these results: López Portillo (460) used *B. turicatae* and found an incubation time of 3 to 7 days when the organisms were administered subcutaneously, and about 6 days when the infection was transmitted by the bite of *O. turicata.* Brumpt and Brumpt (124) observed a somewhat wider variation in the incubation period of *B. turicatae* infections: 4 to 19 days. Wheeler (727) fed infected *O. hermsi* on prisoner volunteers and established the incubation period as being 7 days. He himself became infected when the blood of an infected squirrel squirted on him. The incubation time was also 7 days. Thus, the incubation period in artificially infected individuals varied from 3 to 19 days, with a median of 6 or 7 days.

Wynns (740) estimated that the incubation period of relapsing fever in patients with the tick-borne variety in the United States is 7 to 14 days. The shortest period was 2 days, the longest 29. The same average incubation time was observed in Venezuela (573) and Ecuador (443). This period is somewhat longer than that observed in artificial infections and may be due to improper recall by some patients concerning the time of the tick bite, to differences in the various *Borrelia* strains, or to the number of borreliae carried by the individual ticks. Nevertheless, it seems that the average incubation time is between 5 and 9 days. However, especially in tick-borne infections, cases may also appear later, as long as 2 weeks and sometimes 3 weeks after exposure.

The First Attack

Some authors (557, 731) have reported prodromal symptoms such as headache lasting a few days, weakness, malaise, vertigo, undefined aches and pains, perhaps also vomiting. Prodromes are seldom observed in the Americas (460, 464).

The onset is usually sudden. This was seen in China in 91.5% of the patients in louse-borne (176) as well as in tick-borne infections (93). The same observation has also been registered in other outbreaks and isolated instances.

The onset is usually accompanied by chills. This was observed in 90% of the patients in Villa Nador (503). During the attack, the body temperature usually ranges from 38.7 to 40° C (102° to 104° F), sometimes even 41° C (106° F) (429, 553). The fever lasts 3 to 13 days, on the average 4 to 7 days (282) or 5 to 7 days (388, 664) in the louse-borne form; 3 to 5 days in tick-borne disease (303, 464, 475, 739). Sometimes the temperature reaches its maximum in 24 hours, ascending more slowly. The fever is most often continuous with slight variations. The daily fluctuations, however, may be as much as 3° C (5.5° F). Sometimes, as in the Moroccan louse-borne epidemic (503) and in East and West Africa (467), a precritical rise in the temperature to 41° C (106° F) or less accompanied by profuse sweating, shivering, and even collapse may be observed. The attack ends with a crisis which will be discussed separately. The crisis lasts 1 to 2 hours, or somewhat longer. If the attack ends with a lysis, the course is 1 to 3 days. A typical fever course was seen in China in 96.8% of the patients observed by Jouveau-Dubreuhil (387) but this has been an infrequent finding in other instances.

The pulse rate is usually 110 to 120/min. However, it may show a broader range and wider variations (476). Except in the so-called "bilious" form, the pulse rate is comparable to the body temperature.

Violent occipital or occipito-frontal headache is the leading complaint. It is probably due to increased intracranial pressure. This symptom was emphasized in the World War II epidemic (298), in 90% of the patients with tick-borne infections in Iran (740), and in the louse-borne Abadan outbreak (87). Similar observations were made in 76.2% of the patients in North China by Chung and Chang (176), and others. Headache was not marked, however, in the Qetta episode (114).

Pain and tenderness of the muscles, especially the calves, are considered typical of the disease (205). Others (303) noted pain in the neck. Backache was the principal complaint in 77% of the patients in Iran (87). Sometimes it radiates into the limbs. General aches were reported in 58.5% of the patients in North China (176).

A macular eruption is often seen, consisting of rose-colored spots spreading from the neck to the shoulders, then to the sides of the thorax, to the inner aspects of the thighs and the arms. This rash usually appears at the end of the first paroxysm. The spots may last 1 or 2 days or only a few hours (303, 551). In Abyssinia, it is rather common and either covers most of the skin or remains localized (608). Bryceson *et al.* (127) observed it in 17% of their patients. The rash was rare in Abadan (87) and absent in Qetta (114). In the Asian U.S.S.R. (551) a rash was seen only in 15% of the patients. It appeared shortly before the crisis of the first attack. In Texas, the eruption was described in about 50% of the patients, in other parts of the United States in about 4% (464). The eruption becomes petechial in severe cases. It was often hemorrhagic in Mozambique (469). In North China, a petechial rash was seen in 34.7% of the patients (176), while during the louse-borne outbreak in Morocco it was recorded in about 25%, according to Moreno Berdugo and Infante Gómez (503), who noted that petechial hemorrhages were rather common during the entire World War II louse-borne epidemic but appeared only shortly before the crisis in the World War I (551) outbreak.

Of other hemorrhagic phenomena, hematuria is rare but epistaxis has often been seen in North China, South Africa, and Peru (164). It is more frequent at the end of the first attack (557). Metrorrhagia and melena have also been reported but seem to be rare.

The gastrointestinal tract is frequently involved. Nausea and vomiting are usually present in about one-half of the cases in louse-borne epidemics (176, 620) and often in *B. duttonii* infections (303). The complaints may persist into the apyrexial period (647). They often appear only during the first attack (475) or only during relapses (557), or they may be entirely absent (6). Violent epigastric pain was reported in the louse-borne outbreak in Eritrea by Lanzo and Tresca (432) who called this complex of symptoms "pseudodysentery." These symptoms, as well as many others, depend on vasomotor disturbances and their sequelae and may vary from one instance to another.

Diarrhea may appear during the crisis (647) but it seems to be restricted to certain epidemics. It was rare in louse-borne relapsing fever in Spain, but frequent in Venezuela (573), and present in 14% of the patients in Northern China (175). Diarrhea might be the result of a secondary infection, as in Korea (17).

Constipation has been recorded in borreliosis (154). In North China, as many as 47.4% of the patients with this infection suffered from constipation. It is not known what treatment, if any, could have caused this condition.

The liver may or may not be enlarged. Bryceson *et al.* (127) found it enlarged or tender in 63% of the patients in Addis Ababa. Mild cases seldom show appreciable liver enlargement but this is a frequent finding in severe outbreaks (176, 464). Hepatomegaly was observed in 18% of the patients with *B. hispanica* infections (476). Others (93, 303) also emphasized painful liver. In South Africa, where the number of relapses is usually high in tick-borne relapsing fever, the liver becomes enlarged during relapses (557) and jaundice may also develop. Others, however, seldom observed enlarged liver in moderate or mild cases (114, 432, 460). Thus it appears that the liver is enlarged in serious cases or after several relapses.

Jaundice is frequent in relapsing fever in Abyssinia and accompanies pressure-sensitive liver also in Dakar (97). It was recorded in 29.4% of the patients in North China. A slight jaundice is often observed in African cases (71, 149). The time of onset of the icterus varies. It frequently appears on the third day of the attack, if it develops at all (573). While icterus does not point to a bad prognosis in patients in Peru and Cyprus (242), it is a serious indicator in Iran, China, and East Africa. The "bilious typhoid" of the old literature seems to be relapsing fever with liver involvement (731, 732). Icterus is difficult to see in dark-skinned persons. There may be only an icteric tint of the sclerae. Bryceson *et al.* (127) observed jaundice in 34% of their patients with the louse-borne form, di Benedetto (74) in nearly all cases in East Africa.

The spleen may be enlarged and tender (647) but it becomes smaller between attacks. Splenomegaly has been found in 34.7% of the patients in North China (176), in 10% in Eritrea (432), in 50% in both *B. recurrentis* (127) and *B. hispanica* infections

(467), in 33% of the cases in Texas (464), in 18% but only as a transient phenomenon in Mozambique (469), in nearly all instances in South Africa (557), and irregularly in other areas. Splenomegaly has seldom been seen in relapsing fever in the U.S.S.R. It was absent in Morocco (503) and in other parts of North Africa (467) except when complications such as malaria were simultaneously present. Splenic infarcts were found in 2.5% of the patients, mostly in males, even as early as during the first attack, in Egypt (595).

The size of the spleen, therefore, is not pathognomonic in relapsing fever.

Urinary tract involvements, such as nephritis, have been reported in Tobruk (201) and other areas, but the evidence that these were the result of relapsing fever is not satisfactory. Oliguria was observed in 25.2% of the patients in North China (176). Albuminuria has been found in the majority of the patients in East Africa (74) but rarely in the southern parts of Africa and in North America (see chapter on Pathology).

Respiratory symptoms are frequently observed in relapsing fever (156) also in the United States. Bronchitis and bronchopneumonia have been reported in 60% of the patients in Abadan (87) but only in 16.6% in Egypt by Omar (552). Respiratory symptoms are rare in Eritrea and Israel. Saddle-back temperature curves have been observed when bronchitis has developed during a relapsing fever attack (557). Cough was recorded in about one-half of the patients in Abyssinia but seldom in *B. duttonii* infections (590).

Respiratory symptoms are so frequent in some relapsing fever epidemics that they are often considered part and parcel of the disease proper rather than complications. Cough may be due, however, to hemodynamic changes in the lungs and to secondary infections (127).

Neuropsychiatric symptoms are more common in tick-borne disease than in the louse-borne epidemics. Nevertheless, Bryceson *et al.* (127) recorded meningeal symptoms in 30% of *B. recurrentis* infections. Insomnia is the rule. Tactile and taste hyperesthesias have been recorded by Simmons (647). Meningeal and central nervous system hemorrhages have been reported. Hemiplegias and aphasia have been observed, supposedly resulting from transient nerve defects caused by increased intracranial pressure or bleeding. Meningeal symptoms are not infrequent in the United States (183) and in Spain (390). The spinal fluid contains an increased number of lymphocytes and its pressure is elevated (454). Pre-existing thiamine deficiency may be a predisposing factor for neuritis. On the other hand, the development of "wet" beri-beri has been observed after relapsing fever (180). Post-infectious neuritis may be ascribed to B-vitamin deficiency, principally in borderline nutritional states.

A fatal meningeal form has been described in Ecuador (443). In Africa, either gross central nervous system disturbances, such as aphasia and hemiplegia, are seen, or there may be involvement of specific nerves. Facial paralysis, sometimes of permanent nature, has been described (335). The neurotropic manifestations are transient and usually disappear in about 6 weeks (517). After about the same period after onset in *B. hispanica* infections, 3% of the patients developed paresis, but this cleared up in 3 to 4 weeks (620). Transverse myelitis is seldom seen. Epileptiform seizures have been reported (469), sometimes appearing simultaneously with neuralgia and neuritis.

If permanent paralysis develops, it is mostly that of the facial nerve (635). Encephalitic damage in relapsing fever has a tendency to remain stationary.

Psychoneurotic symptoms are frequent in patients in Syria and Lebanon (625), Kenya (296), Central Africa (454), Madagascar (517), North Africa (31), South Africa (633), and Poland (453), but they are less common in Dakar (93) and Abyssinia (156). They are rare in the United States. They may appear late, 2 to 2½ months after the onset of the disease, as in *B. duttonii* infections (582, 583).

Psychotic phenomena have been classified by Aubin *et al.* (31) as:

(a) Confusional, with terrifying dreams and possible suicidal tendency. This form is quite common.
(b) Anxiety complex, which may develop after a period of confusion. It is often maniacal, rarely depressive, with delusions, irritability, and impulsiveness.
(c) Protracted type, which is rare. Various hallucinatory and delusional forms were noted in this group.

The time of the appearance of psychotic disturbances varies.

They may be noted as early as during the incubation period. When they develop in convalescence, the symptoms tend to be atypical. The history of such patients often shows alcoholism and syphilis in addition to relapsing fever.

Ocular disturbances such as iritis, cyclitis, and chorioiditis have

TABLE 3
SUMMARY OF THE COURSE OF RELAPSING FEVER

	Louse-borne	*Tick-borne*					
		U.S.A.	*So. Amer.*	*Africa@*	*Medi-terran*	*Near East*	*Central Asia*
Incubation period	5-8* (2-15)°	6-7 (2-14, s 14-20)	6-7	2-10 (2-14)	5-9 (4-11)	6-14 (5-18)	6-12 (5-14)
Duration of 1st attack	5-7 (3-13)	3-4 (1-19)	5-9 (1-20)	3-6 (1-10)	2-4 (1-5)	2-6 (1-8)	2-4 (1-6)
First afebrile interval	5-7 (3-9, s m)	3-14 (3-20)	4-15 (4-23)	6-8 (5-14)	7-15 (3-30)	irreg.	irreg.
Duration of subsequent relapses^x	1-4 (1-8)	1-3 (1-5)	1-3 (1-6)	5-6 (4-10)	1-5 (1-10)	irreg.	irreg.
No. of relapses	0-4 (0-10)	0-3 (0-5)	1-5 (3-8)	3-9 (3-20)	1-5 (1-18)	irreg. (0-10)	irreg. (0-20)
Course of disease	V	us. mild	us. moder.	oft. severe	V, oft. mild	oft. severe	V, us. moder.
Rash	+	++	+++	oft. hemorrh.	+	+	+
Icterus	++	V	++	+++	+	+	+
Hepatomegaly	+++	+++	+++	++++	++	++	+
Splenomegaly	+++	++	++	++++	++	+	±
Meningism	+	++	+++	+++	++	++	+
Severe C.N.S. involvement	+	+	++	+++	±	++	±
Extensive hemorrhages	+	±	+	++♯	±	±	±

@ East, West and So. Africa
* usual length, in days
° range, in days
s seldom
m more
x if any
V variable
♯ mostly in So. Africa

± in less than 10% of the patients
\+ in 10 to 25% of the patients
++ in 25 to 40% of the patients
+++ in 40 to 80% of the patients
++++ in more than 80% of the patients

often been described (335, 469); these have a good prognosis. Conjunctivitis is common in South America and South Africa. Iridocyclitis is an important manifestation, having been observed in 3% of patients with *B. hispanica* infections. It persists for 2 to 3 weeks (476). It has also been observed in about 14% of the patients in East Africa. It is rare in the United States but frequently described in Madagascar (517). Hamilton (335) did not see ophthalmic lesions in Syria, but these were present in about 20% of his patients in the Western Desert of Africa. Both acute and chronic iridocyclitis were observed. The iridocyclitis may lead to synechiae which are easily broken down by mydriatics. This author (335) did not see chorioiditis but observed a gross vitreous exudate. The affection was unilateral and the prognosis for the vision was good. Chorioiditis was encountered, however, in both Cyprus (738) and Mozambique (469). Ophthalmia due to treatment with arsenicals was common during the World War II epidemic (298).

In Romania (205), middle ear infections ascending from the nasopharynx were reported in 70% of the patients. This complication is rare at present.

Different hematologic pictures have been reported from various areas. These have been discussed in the chapter on Pathology. Here we would like to record that Whitmore (731) noted a progressive anemia with a decrease in the red blood cell count and hemoglobin. This was seen also in louse-borne disease in Morocco, Spain, and China (388), and in tick-borne relapsing fever in Madagascar (672). In Madagascar, polychromasia and some poikilocytosis were also noted. A hemolytic tendency with the appearance of young red blood cells in the peripheral blood has been recorded in East Africa (67). Little hematologic response has been manifest either along the Mediterranean, in the U.S.S.R., or in the United States.

The platelet count is low (127).

The total number of white blood cells increases to 15,000 to 26,000 according to Simmons (647), but Whitmore (731) reported only a moderate leukocytosis. Variable counts have been reported by Beeson (71), from Israel (419), from the U.S.S.R., and the Western Mediterranean (503). A substantial leukocytosis was considered a bad prognostic sign in China (163). Leukocytosis is frequently noted during bronchitis and when the fever rises.

The white cell count may be normal or elevated during the attacks as well as in the afebrile periods. This was seen in World War I (482), and was probably due to secondary infections. The number of leukocytes may be high during the attacks but it is low during remissions. A shift of the neutrophiles to the left is usually observed, especially while *Borrelia* persists in the body (482).

TABLE 4
SUMMARY OF CLINICAL PATHOLOGIC FINDINGS
DURING FEBRILE PERIODS

Hemoglobin	very often decreased, principally during relapses
Red blood cells	frequently decreased
White blood cells	frequently increased but decreased before crisis in louse-borne, variable in tick-borne. If elevated during afebrile periods, sign of secondary infection
Shift to the left	very frequent, persists when attack will be repeated and in secondary infections
Eosinopenia	very frequent, except in helminthic infections
Lymphocytosis	frequent during attack, principally before crisis but often variable
Monocytosis	very frequent, may decrease just before febrile episode
Blood platelets	very frequently decreased
Red blood cell sedimentation rate	very frequently increased
Prothrombin time	frequently prolonged
Bleeding time	rarely prolonged
Clotting time	very frequently prolonged
Blood urea N	frequently increased
Plasma Cl	frequently decreased
Serum bilirubin	less frequently increased
Serum transaminases	frequently increased
Serum alkaline phosphatase	frequently increased
Total serum protein	sometimes increased
Serum gamma globulins	very frequently increased
Urinary protein	very frequently present, less often in the U.S.A.
Urine bile pigments	very frequently increased
Red blood cells in urine	frequently increased, very frequently increased in Africa

There is a decrease in the eosinophil count (234, 621). This may be the only abnormality in the blood picture (437). The number of eosinophils may be low only during attacks, especially if eosinophilia caused by parasites is present during afebrile periods (387). The number of lymphocytes may be increased during the attacks, especially during the crisis according to most observers, but it may fluctuate.

Monocytosis was the only change in the blood picture observed in Qetta (114). The monocyte count was increased during the World War I epidemic. In the region of the Chad in Africa, monocytes comprised as much as 60% of the white blood cells in the World War II epidemic (439). The number often increases in tick-borne disease (590).

The monocyte count often decreases before the onset of symptoms and increases during the relapse, reaching its maximum just at the beginning of the interval between relapses.

The sedimentation rate of the red blood cells is increased (744). Prothrombin deficiency has been noted in louse-borne relapsing fever in patients in Addis Ababa (127, 608).

The blood picture changes with the phases of the disease and, perhaps, also with the infectious agent.

Cardiac difficulties are seldom encountered in the United States. The electrocardiogram (ECG) has been normal in the examined cases (404). Abnormal ECG has been observed in louse-borne borreliosis (127), particularly a prolonged Q-Tc interval. Cardiac murmurs indicative of valvular endocarditis have been reported (607). Endocarditis and myocarditis, confirmed at autopsy, have been related by several authors (296, 475, 557 and others).

There usually is tachycardia during the attack, with a pulse rate of 100 to 140 per minute (460, 476). Tachypnea is the rule, with 28 to 42 respirations per minute.

Other symptoms are congested, but dry, face (476); furred tongue with red edges and a brown coating similar to that seen in typhus; and frequently abdominal pain and tenderness. Lymph node enlargement has also been noted at times.

It is often difficult or impossible to find the place of the tick bite on the skin of the patient. Louse-infested patients usually show many traces of insect bites.

Duration of the First Attack

As stated above, the initial attack in the louse-borne type lasts 3 to 13 days, on the average 4 to 7 days, according to the epidemic (453). In Abyssinia, it now lasts 4 to 10 days (127). In the Darjeeling outbreak (392), the first attack terminated after 8 to 10 days and there were no relapses. Such irregularities have been observed also in later epidemics (732).

The duration of the initial attack in tick-borne relapsing fever was recorded as 3 hours to 4 days in Palestine (6), as one day, seldom 3 to 4 days in the U.S.S.R. (398, 655), 2 to 4 days in Africa (557), and 9 hours to 9 days (usually 3 days) in the United States (464). Considerable variations were observed in *B. persica* infections (739). Thus the duration of the first attack of tick-borne relapsing fever is usually shorter than that of louse-borne borreliosis.

The Crisis

Crisis follows the partial or total disintegration of the borreliae in the circulation. There is a sudden, abrupt drop in the temperature, often to subnormal, accompanied by low blood pressure, intensive sweating, and weakness. The patient may go into shock. Convulsions due to cerebral edema or thrombosis, and myocardial failure may set in.

After the crisis, many patients feel weak. The further course of the disease depends on several factors, among which are the causative agent, the resistance of the host, and a number of unknown elements often designated as the "*genius epidemicus*".

The Interval

There may be only one attack. In other instances, the body temperature, pulse rate, and blood pressure may remain subnormal or the patient may have no complaints or clinical symptoms until the relapse occurs.

The interval between the first attack and the subsequent first relapse varies. In louse-borne relapsing fever it may be 5 to 9 (664), usually 5 to 6 days (127). It was 3 to 16 days (176) in China, and 7 days (298) during the World War II epidemic. In tick-borne borreliosis this interval is irregular but usually lasts one week (303), 4 to 15 days in South America, is irregular in Iran, and lasts 3 to 36 days in the United States (464).

Relapses

As a general rule, in louse-borne fever the relapses occur at shorter intervals than in the tick-borne disease (215, 647), but not in South America (460 and others). Relapses have a tendency to become shorter and milder as the disease gradually abates.

There is considerable variation, however, in the course of the illness, especially in epidemics. In Africa (298, 323), Europe (297 and others), and in China before World War I and during the World War II outbreak, only one relapse was observed in the majority of patients with louse-borne relapsing fever. About 5% had more than two relapses, with a maximum of 5. Relapses were more frequent in North China. In Abyssinia, up to 4 relapses are often seen (127). The interval between the relapses averaged 7 days in China, with a minimum of 3 and a maximum of 16 days. The duration of the relapses was 2 to 10 days, averaging 5 days. The time interval between the relapses was 7½ to 11 days in the Abadan outbreak, each relapse lasting 2½ to 5 days (87).

Relapsing fever carried by ticks usually shows many relapses, especially in Asia and in Africa. There are significant individual variations, however, (123, 739), which make the prediction of the course of an individual case difficult. Three to 5 relapses should be expected on the average. Their number may be more in Central Asia, up to 20 (398, 655). In Central Africa, usually 5 to 12 relapses, each lasting 5 to 6 days, occur (303). In the Americas, the patients fall in equal percentages into each of the following categories: no relapse, 1 relapse, 2 relapses, 3 relapses, and more than 3 relapses. *B. turicatae* infections, as well as borreliae of the crocidurae subgroup, cause few or no relapses. Three to 5 relapses, each lasting less than 3 days, have been described (60). The interval between the initial attack and the first relapse varies from 3 to 40 days, and the duration of the first and subsequent relapses from a few hours to not more than 4 days.

Thus louse-borne relapsing fever is usually milder than tick-borne, with short and few (1 or 2, maximum 6) relapses. The tick-borne variety is more severe and prolonged. The number of relapses during this form of the disease generally varies from 2 to 5 in America and the Mediterranean area; in some infections in Central Asia and Central Africa as many as 10 to 22 relapses are often observed (303, 685, 731).

The total course of the untreated louse-borne relapsing fever is short, 1 to 2 weeks. Untreated tick-borne disease may last 3 weeks to 7 months (625).

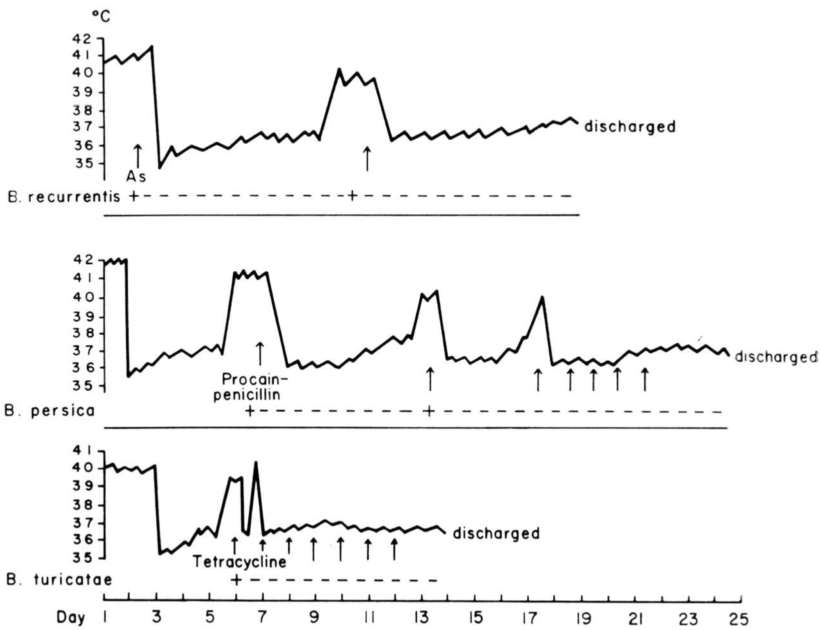

FIGURE 30. Fever curves of patients infected with various *Borrelia* strains.

Illustrative Case Histories

1. This patient was seen in China in 1933.

W.C.-L., a slightly built Chinese housekeeper, 52-year-old mother of 3 children, was brought to the hospital with complaints of fever and chills, nausea and vomiting, pain in the abdomen of indefinite location, and dry cough. The patient was apathetic, with a flushed face, and an icteric tint of the sclerae. The tongue was brown with clean edges. There were stridor and some rales audible at the base of the lungs. The liver extended about 6 to 7 cm below the costal margin in the parasternal line, and was sensitive on palpation. The abdomen was tender over the colon and also around the umbilicus. The spleen did not appear enlarged on physical examination. The temperature was 40.8° C, the pulse rate 110 per minute, the blood pressure 110/65 mm Hg. There was lethargy, some nuchal rigidity, diminished abdominal reflexes, and pain in the limbs on palpation.

Blood, spinal fluid, urine, and stools were collected for laboratory tests.

The next day the sensorium remained unchanged. Vomiting ceased. The sclerae were suffused and remained icteric. The rales persisted over the lungs. The patient complained of backache and pain in the legs. The liver was more tender than on the previous day but its margin did not appear altered. The spleen was soft and tender. Nuchal rigidity persisted. The temperature remained elevated.

The laboratory reported increased urobilinogen in the urine, no sugar, 2+ protein, a positive benzidine reaction, few hyaline casts, but only rare red blood cells. Total serum protein was 8 Gm%, blood urea 55 mg%, and blood sugar 87 mg%. The icterus index was 14. The spinal fluid showed 15 cells per cu.mm, 42 mg% glucose, 68 mg% protein. Hematologic examination revealed 3.9 million red blood cells, 11,000 white blood cells, 9.9 Gm% hemoglobin, and a differential white cell count of 18% juveniles, 30% segmented neutrophils, less than 1% eosinophils and basophils, 13% monocytes, and 39% lymphocytes. The erythrocytic sedimentation rate was 105 mm per hour.

Agglutination tests with *Proteus OX19, OXK,* and typhoid antigen were negative. Malarial parasites were not found in the blood films but borreliae were present. A diagnosis was therefore made of borreliosis, or relapsing fever.

The patient was given 40 mg Mapharsen intravenously, and 15 mg codein t.i.d., the latter to alleviate the pain.

The next day the temperature fell abruptly to 34.8° C. The pulse rate was 100 per minute. The blood pressure dropped to 70/40 mm Hg. The patient was drenched with sweat. Petechial hemorrhages appeared over the trunk and upper limbs. According to the practice prevailing at that time, adrenalin was administered.

During the subsequent 6 days, the patient appeared very weak.

The hemorrhagic spots disappeared progressively. Lack of appetite, and some pain in the lower limbs persisted. Nuchal rigidity was not apparent, and the deep muscular reflexes were normal. The liver and spleen returned to approximately normal size. Borreliae were not found in the blood that was examined daily. On the seventh day after the first attack, the patient suddenly developed chills, the temperature rose to 39.8° C, the eyes became bloodshot, the face flushed and dry. Borreliae reappeared in the blood stream. There was some hesitation to repeat the administration of the arsenical because it was not certain whether the hemorrhagic phenomena were due to the usual course of the disease or were part of a reaction to Mapharsen. The fever continued, splenic enlargement became more accentuated, and signs of meningeal irritation developed, including a positive Kernig's phenomenon. Mapharsen was therefore repeated, 30 mg intravenously. This was followed by an abrupt fall in the temperature. The pulse rate was 80 per minute. The sweating was profuse but there were no hemorrhagic phenomena. The liver did not become enlarged. The blood picture showed 8,000 white blood cells, 3.5 million red blood cells, 8.9 Gm% hemoglobin. Recovery was uneventful, except for a feeling of weakness. Borreliae were not seen again in the blood films. The patient was discharged 7 days later.

The causative organism was classified as *Borrelia recurrentis* in cross-protection tests in mice against the Chinese type strain.

The patient appeared to be in an adequate physical condition before discharge. The spinal fluid protein was 12 mg%, glucose 42 mg%, the cell count 3 per cu.mm. The urine did not show increased urobilinogen, and tests for protein and sugar were negative. There were a few hyaline casts and leukocytes in the sediment. The blood urea was 20 mg%; the serum icterus index 4. There were 6,000 white blood cells per cu.mm. The differential count was juveniles 6%, polymorphonuclear neutrophils 60%, eosinophils and basophils 2%, monocytes 8%, lymphocytes 24%. The red blood cell count was 3.3 million cells per cu.mm.; Hb 8.7 Gm%. Treatment with iron preparations was recommended, and the patient was transferred to the clinic.

2. This patient was seen in Afghanistan in 1948.

A.M.E.H., a well-built Afghan male sheepherder, 24 years old, single, living with a group that had been moving with their livestock, and sleeping under tents or in caves.

He was admitted to the hospital with 42° C fever, pulse rate 140/min, flushed face, a few roseolae on the abdomen, and complaining of headache and pain in the back. The spleen was moderately enlarged and painful on palpation. There was no jaundice. The liver was within limits considered normal. There were conjunctivitis and photophobia. The abdomen was not tender, except for the left upper quadrant. Physical examination did not reveal other abnormalities. The urine analysis report was specific gravity 1.032; no sugar or casts, but protein was present. The blood films were negative for parasites. The tentative diagnosis was F.U.O. (fever of unknown origin), perhaps smallpox, and the patient was put into isolation.

The temperature suddenly decreased to 35.7° C the next day. The patient was sweating profusely. The pulse rate was 65 per minute. He was restless and complained more of thirst than of pain. Later after the abrupt fall in the temperature the patient felt well. Daily blood film examinations did not reveal parasites. Bacteriologic cultures of the stools were not indicative of a *Salmonella* infection. Blood cultures remained negative. On the fourth day after the crisis, the patient developed chills and high fever. The blood films revealed borreliae. A diagnosis was therefore made of relapsing fever. He was given 500,000 units of procaine penicillin intramuscularly. Shortly thereafter a crisis took place. It was believed that the patient was on the road of recovery, when 5 days later the temperature again reached 40.1° C. Procaine penicillin was repeated in the same dosage. The temperature dropped abruptly, and the patient remained symptomless for 3 days, when the temperature rose somewhat more slowly to 39.8° C, and borreliae again appeared in the blood. Thereafter procaine penicillin was repeated daily for 5 consecutive days, 500,000 units per day. The proteinuria disappeared at that time. There were no subjective complaints. The spleen became smaller and was no longer tender. The patient was discharged 6 days after the last relapse.

The meager laboratory studies of this case were due to the inadequate facilities available at the local hospital. The organisms were tested in the Pasteur Institute of Teheran and classified as *B. persica*.

It does not seem that penicillin in the doses administered was of much value in this case.

3. This patient was seen in Thailand in 1958.

A.S.B. was an American boy, 11 years old, somewhat overweight, who had returned with his parents from home-leave in Texas. There he had romped in the woods around their home until the day before the family returned by fast air transportation to Bangkok. A few days later he developed fever and chills, vomited several times, started coughing, and complained of severe headache and pain in the chest and in the limbs. On admission to the hospital, his face was dry and flushed, the conjunctivae were injected, and the muscles of the abdomen and the limbs were tender. The rest of the physical examination did not reveal any deviations from the normal. Chest x-rays and the results of urine examinations were negative. Tests on the serum showed 11 mg% Ca, 605 mg% Na as NaCl, 31 mg% urea, 8.1 Gm% protein (albumin: globulin ratio 1.3:1). Plasma fibrinogen was 170 mg%. The prothrombin time was 13 seconds, the coagulation time (glass tube method) 17 minutes, the hematocrit value 38 ml%. Hematologic studies revealed 12.8 Gm% hemoglobin, 4.6 million red blood cells, 120,-000 platelets, and 5,000 white blood cells per cu.mm. There were 10% juvenile neutrophils, 24% segmented neutrophils, less than 1% eosinophils and basophils, 58% lymphocytes, and 18% monocytes. The tourniquet test showed 4 petechiae in a 5 cm circle after 5 minutes with the cuff at 100 mm Hg pressure. Blood, urine, and stool cultures were negative. No malarial parasites were found in the blood films.

The tentative diagnosis was fever of unknown origin, perhaps dengue fever. Blood specimens were submitted for virologic examination. The patient received aspirin which reduced the pain but did not influence the course of the fever. He was also given 5% glucose infusions with B-vitamin complex. On the third day the patient was apathetic, and a papular exanthem appeared on the flexor surfaces of the arms, spreading distally but disappearing after 6 to 7 hours. Then the patient started sweating, and the temperature fell from 40.4° C to 35.5° C within a few hours. The pulse rate decreased from 135 to 65 per minute, and the blood pressure dropped from 105/75 to 70/40 mm Hg. The patient felt better, and the temperature as well as the blood pressure began to return to normal. Pains and aches appeared again on the third day after the crisis. Chills and fever returned, just at the time when young mice inoculated with the patient's blood collected during the first attack showed borreliae in their circulation. A thorough check of the blood films collected during the second episode also revealed these organisms. A diagnosis was made of relapsing fever.

Tetracycline was given, 0.1 Gm parenterally. An immediate critical drop in the temperature was observed followed by a brief rise to 40.3° C. The borreliae disappeared from the blood, and after drenching sweat for a few hours, the pains subsided and the patient appeared to become interested in his environment, responsive, thirsty, and hungry. It was decided, therefore, to maintain tetracycline medication at a low level for 6 more days, administering per os 0.25 Gm twice a day. Recovery was uneventful. The organisms were diagnosed as *B. turicatae* by immobilizine and borreliolysin tests using antisera against *B. turicatae, B. parkerii,* and *B. hermsii.*

At discharge, the patient had no complaints. Chest x-ray, E.C.G., urine, and spinal fluid examinations showed no deviations from the normal for his age. The blood serum showed 12 mg% Ca, 585 mg% Na as NaCl, 28 mg% urea, 6.5 Gm% protein (albumin: globulin ratio 1.4:1). Plasma fibrinogen was 240 mg%. The icterus index was 4. The prothrombin time was 12 seconds, the coagulation time 15 minutes, the hematocrit value 40 ml%. Hematologic studies revealed 12.3 Gm% hemoglobin, 4.2 millon red blood cells, 210,000 platelets, and 7,000 white blood cells per cu.mm. There were 3% juvenile neutrophils, 42% segmented neutrophils, 3% eosinophils, 1% basophils, 45% lymphocytes, and 6% monocytes. The tourniquet test showed no petechiae.

It was possible to obtain serum samples from this patient also after convalescence. There was an increase of the immobilizine titer from less than 5% in the sera collected during the attacks to 53% and 61%, respectively, one and three months after discharge from the hospital. The borreliocidin titers reached 1:360 at the same time. Cross-reactions with cardiolipin were not observed but a serum sample collected during the second attack gave an agglutinin titer of 1:40 with *Proteus OXK* but not with *Proteus OX19.*

The temperature curves of these patients are shown in Fig. 30.

Atypical Forms

The temperature curve may show aberrations. In tick-borne cases in Iran, variations have been recorded from mild fever for a few days without relapses to severe disease with irregular temperatures for 14 to 16 days, followed by irregular spiking remissions (739). Long paroxysms of continuous low-grade fever were also seen in the Mediterranean area.

Very mild, ambulatory but protracted tick-borne cases have been reported from the Southeastern Mediterranean (419, 420), contrasting with fulminating disease that killed the patient within 24 hours, in Africa (467).

Atypical forms have been grouped according to the predominant clinical syndromes by several authors, as in Abyssinia (240), in North Africa (395), and in Ecuador (443). These forms may be summarized as ambulatory, dysenteriform, typhoid-like, hepatic, biliary, pulmonary, meningoencephalitic, and rheumatoid.

Schuhardt (630) explained the different number of relapses by the diverse ability of the various *Borrelia* strains to form antigenic phase variants during the disease to which antibodies are not available as a result of immunologic experience acquired during the previous course of the disease. There is no explanation for the difference in the capability of various strains to form such phases. One may consider them an expression of the antigenic instability of borreliae, which supports the concept that there is only one species of *Borrelia,* and all *Borrelia* types we are speaking and writing about are mere variants of only one single microbial entity. Awareness of these atypical forms is important not only for the clinician but also for the epidemiologist, particularly in the beginning and at the end of epidemics when they appear more frequently.

Complications

Otitis, parotitis, and arthritis have been listed in standard textbooks. Cardiac disturbances frequently occur in the Caucasus, Kenya (296), Abyssinia (127, 608), and in Ecuador (443). In South Africa (557), heart failure and residual arthritis causing "rheumatic" pains have been observed. In addition to circulatory disturbances, hemorrhages, principally in the central nervous system, may cause problems.

Hepatic failure is a serious complication.

Splenic rupture may cause death. More than 90% of pregnant women abort when infected with *Borrelia* (298, 552).

Herpes labialis is frequent, especially in louse-borne infections (503) but may occur also in tick-borne borreliosis with varying frequency (335, 476, 503).

Secondary infections of the respiratory tract are common. Salmonellosis is often a fatal secondary infection (17). Epidemic typhus fever presents a grave menace (734). Latent malaria and kala azar may be activated by relapsing fever (202).

Reinfection

Kudicke *et al.* (427) called attention to the role played by treatment in the development of resistance against reinfection. If the disease has terminated abruptly, before antibodies developed, reinfection with the same strain appears a distinct possibility. Reinfection, however, is rare in louse-borne epidemics if proper hygienic measures are enforced, principally delousing and prevention of reinfestation with ectoparasites. However, reinfection may occur in 2 months according to Simmons (647), in 1½ to 6 months according to Whitmore (731), and in one year according to Más de Ayala (476). In tick-borne infections in Central Asia, Kassirsky (398) observed a shorter period of immunity against reinfections but Grothusen (326) demonstrated that the disease caused by *B. duttonii* in Africans may be as severe as in Europeans who did not have an opportunity to acquire premunition during their childhood. Childhood infection is, however, of paramount importance for the response to a later infection according to other authors (263, 303, 443, 715, 732).

Apparently, recurrence *versus* reinfection should be re-evaluated also in relapsing fever (263).

Hereditary immunity is a moot question. Nohira (546) demonstrated in rats that the offspring of the female infected with *B. recurrentis* is immune to the homologous strain for about 2 months. Women with relapsing fever usually abort and few data are available about infants delivered at term, except in studies of congenital transmission. Such instances were described in the United States (183, 283, 505); by Garnham (1936), Caldwell (1936), Kröber (1936) and Correa *et al.* (1964) in Africa (139, 203, 292, 424); and in other areas (176). Further studies of transplacental antibody transmission are most desirable, principally in regard to the recent concept of immunoglobulins of which only the small-sized IgG appears to be transmitted to the newborn.

Prognosis and Mortality

Sterling-Okunewski (669) demonstrated that the number of borreliae in the peripheral circulation has no bearing on the severity of the disease or on the prognosis of relapsing fever.

Mayer (482) considered continuous high fever, deep jaundice, extensive hemorrhages, and coma as bad prognostic signs. León and León (443) added to this list endocarditis and myocarditis. Bryceson *et al.* (127) called attention also to persistent Q-Tc interval changes in the ECG, disseminated intravascular coagulation. hepatic failure, cerebral edema, and shock as serious prognostic signs. Pneumonia was cause for a bad prognosis in China (176).

The disease frequently has a severe course in infants.

The case fatality rate in louse-borne relapsing fever depends on the nature of the epidemic and on the availability of treatment. The average mortality in Europe was 4 to 5%; however, in China, Indochina, and India before World War II it fluctuated between 25 and 80%, especially in untreated individuals (495, 731). The small but severe outbreaks in Darjeeling (392) and Assam (152) produced many fatalities, while in Iran few treated patients died (337). On the other hand, in Peru, in spite of the lack of intensive medical care, the case mortality rate was below 2% (164).

During World War II when arsenicals were routinely used, only 0.25% of the treated patients failed to recover, whereas in China about 40% of untreated patients died (163). In Abadan, where good medical care was available, the mortality rate was 1.1% (87). Wide variations, from 1 to 46%, were observed in Tunis, varying according to the locality and the available treatment (323).

In the epidemic following World War II, the case fatality rate was 5 to 10% in untreated individuals, 8.5% in the poor, and 3.6% in the well-to-do (298). The mortality rate among children reached 65% in some areas.

Manson and Thornton (467) calculated a case fatality rate of 0.3% in East Africa, and 4% in West Africa. Garnham *et al.* (296) encountered a 40% mortality among the untreated. Geigy (303) reported 0.7 to 70% deaths.

The mortality figures in crocidurae subgroup infections and in patients in Central Asia are low (398). In the Americas, few of the tick-borne infections cause death (137, 740) except in Venezuela where 27% of the patients died (18). Higher rates, up to 5%, have been reported from Africa (577).

The introduction of antibiotics in the treatment of relapsing fever has greatly reduced the mortality rate.

Laboratory Diagnosis

Microscopic examination

The laboratory diagnosis of infection with *Borrelia* is often made during the attack by examining thin and thick blood films. The slides are stained in Giemsa solution in water at pH 7.2 or with the Wright stain, followed by 10 or 30 seconds in a 1% solution of crystal violet.

Thin blood films should be fixed with acetone or methyl alcohol for 3 minutes before the Giemsa stain is used. Thick smears should be dehemoglobinized with 0.5% acetic acid, carefully washed with water at pH 7.2, and stained without fixation. The evaluation of thick smears may cause difficulties to the less experienced technician.

Laboratory workers often prefer to examine blood preparations under dark field illumination. A drop of the patient's blood is placed on a slide, covered with a coverslip, and the coverslip hermetically sealed with liquid paraffin, wax, a mounting medium, or nail polish. Borreliae remain alive; their movement can be observed with ease in such preparations for several hours.

Fluorescent microscopy requires special equipment and antisera (184). It is practical in areas where only few *Borrelia* serotypes have to be considered.

Borreliae may be sparse in the peripheral circulation during attacks, especially in children (139, 365). Borreliae are usually absent from the blood during the periods between relapses.

In tissues, they can be demonstrated by a silver stain, e.g., that of Krajian which is described in the Appendix.

Animal inoculation

The "standard" animals are young mice which are susceptible to all known human relapsing fever strains. They may or may not succumb to the infection but the borreliae will circulate in their blood. Mouse inoculation is also feasible for examination of the C.S.F. The mouse test is considered superior to the examination of slides (90, 92, 338), whereas Gönnert and Mudrow-Reichenau (320) prefer microscopy to animal experimentations. Chohan (166) recently reemphasized that injecting mice with blood of patients gives better diagnostic results than examining blood films. He studied *O. tholozani*-borne relapsing fever in Kashmir. Only 15.2% of the blood films in clinically ill individuals revealed borreliae. The organisms did appear, however, in the blood stream of the mice 2 to 3 days after inoculation with the patients' blood, and remained in the circulation for 3 to 4 days. This author isolated borreliae from the patients blood with the aid of mouse inoculation also during the apyrexial period.

Usually, 6 to 8 young mice are inoculated intraperitoneally, each with 1 to 2 ml blood of the patient. Borrelemia appears in 2 to 3 days as a rule but it is good practice to examine the blood of the mice for a week before considering it negative. The blood is collected by clipping the end of the tail of the mouse and is examined by dark field illumination or after staining according to Wright or Giemsa.

When mice are inoculated with spinal fluid, 0.5 to 1 ml amounts may have to be injected, and the number of mice reduced if only insufficient amounts of C.S.F. are available.

Mice do not often have relapses. Young rats have also been used but borreliae sometimes suddenly disappear from their blood, even though relapses may be observed in them.

Xenodiagnosis

Baltazard *et al.* (51) applied xenodiagnosis, with good results. The use of *O. moubata* was recently recommended for this purpose by Geigy (303). Five to 10 ticks are fed on the patient during the febrile period and specimens of the hemolymph are examined after a few weeks following aspiration with a capillary tube (129).

An absolute prerequisite for this test is that a tick colony free from borreliae and other infections and infestations be at hand.

Serologic Tests

Serologic tests are seldom helpful during the first days of the disease.

Schuhardt (630) and Felsenfeld (264) summarized the tests used in the serologic diagnosis of *Borrelia* infections, the difficulties due to phase variations of the infective strains in the patient, and the disadvantages inherent in such tests. Production of sufficient amounts of antigen is toilsome because the organisms cannot be easily grown in laboratory culture media.

Agglutination

The value of the agglutination tests is hampered by the natural tendency of the borreliae toward autoagglutination. Balteanu *et al.* (65) were able, however, to demonstrate rising agglutinin titers after attacks.

In our hands, the method of Turner for leptospirae (693) gave good results if adherence could be avoided. Organisms were isolated from rat blood after hemolysis with distilled water at pH 7.2, then centrifuged for 30 minutes at 6,000 r.p.m., and then treated with neutral formol to give a final concentration of 0.2%. The slide method was employed, using 0.01 ml of the antigen, and an equal volume of two-fold serum dilutions. The slides were sealed hermetically, incubated at 37° C for 2 hours, then examined at ×100 magnification by darkfield illumination. We do not recommend this procedure for routine use.

Adhesin Test

The adhesin test has been recommended by Brussin (125) and Schuhardt (360).

The adhesin tests is carried out by mixing serial serum dilutions, a suspension of borreliae, and an *Escherichia coli* suspension, incubating for 20 minutes at 30° C, and then reading the results by darkfield illumination. Adhesion of the borreliae to the *E. coli* organisms can be seen if the test is "positive." Schuhardt (630) observed that a particulate substance does not have to be added if defibrinated nonreactive blood is mixed with the examined serum and the *Borrelia* suspension.

The adhesin test is difficult to replicate and is, therefore, seldom carried out.

Complement Fixation

The complement fixation test was advocated by Toyoda (688).

Complement fixation gives low titers (up to 1:100) either with saponin-treated blood of infected rats (688) or with phenolized egg-grown antigen (737).

The technic of Wolstenhome and Gear (737) consists of inoculating developing chick embryos with mouse blood, harvesting the borreliae one week later after bleeding from the allantoic veins into the allantoic fluid, and passaging this embryonic blood-*Borrelia* mixture ten times through fertilized chicken eggs. The final harvest is taken up in 0.5% phenol-saline, centrifuged, and the supernate used as the antigen. At least 100 borreliae per oil immersion field are necessary for the preparation of a good antigen.

Considerable cross-reaction between the strains, and anticomplementary phenomena frequently mar this test.

Borreliolysin

Several authors (43, 65, 72, 136, 262, 572, 630 and others) have found the borreliolysin test valuable. For instance, Balteanu *et al.* (65) found titers up to 1:1,000 after attacks. Ballif *et al.* (43) stated that high borreliolysin levels may be found as early as during the crisis in *B. recurrentis* infections. Borreliolysin titers up to 1:20,000 have been observed. Pfister (572) reported excellent results employing this test in relapsing fevers caused by *B. hispanica.* Lysin-fast variants may develop, however (132), which do not react in this test.

The borreliolysin test may be carried out with fresh serum to which an equal amount of a standardized suspension of borreliae in physiologic saline is added. Schuhardt (630) recommended that serum and antigen be drawn into a small capillary tube, with a rubber bulb at one end. The contents of the capillary are expelled on an ordinary microscope slide or into a welled slide, mixed, then redrawn into the capillary. The capillary is sealed with wax or clay, incubated at 37° C for 2 hours, the sealed end is broken, and the contents are emptied onto a slide. The number of borreliae are counted under darkfield illumination and compared with the number of organisms in the control, which contains an equal amount of physiologic saline instead of serum.

Balteanu *et al.* (65) found that treatment of the patient may interfere with the test. The borreliolytic activity of the serum persists unchanged in refrigerated serum for 10 months. These authors also used dried blood samples for the test.

Borreliolysin is complement-dependent (265, 268). We, therefore, add guinea pig complement diluted 1:100. Diluting fluids that are supplied with some commercially available desiccated complement contain a preservative, e.g., sodium azide, and cannot be used to reconstitute the dehydrated complement if it is to be employed in this test. The complement is diluted instead with 0.01 M phosphate buffer, containing 5 mM calcium chloride, pH 7.2.

Slides or microplates that fit under a microscope can be used for the test. Our standard *Borrelia* suspensions contain 20 to 30 organisms per high power field. An equal part of serum, inactivated at 56° C for 30 minutes, is mixed with live *Borrelia* suspension. After 30 minutes at 37° C, one part of the diluted complement is added. After 90 minutes further incubation at 37° C, the number of surviving borreliae are counted and compared with the controls. One control contains one part of the *Borrelia* suspension and two parts of physiologic saline, the other equal parts of physiologic saline, *Borrelia* suspension, and diluted complement.

Aliquots of 0.02, 0.025, or 0.05 ml of each component are used. Desiccation must be prevented during incubation. Keeping the slides in a "moist chamber" with a wet piece of filter paper on the bottom will serve this purpose.

The reaction may be carried out in tests tubes, using larger amounts of the reactants. Adequate samples are transferred from the tubes, with an automatic pipette, to slides for microscopic examination.

It is recommended that the borreliae be counted in at least 10 fields, and the results expressed in per cent of organisms lysed. For instance, if 300 organisms were counted in the control and 120 in the slide containing the examined serum, 180 borreliae were lysed, i.e., 60%, which is the titer of the serum.

Schuhardt (630) stated that *immobilizines* may or may not be related to lysins. Our group (264, 265, 268) reported that immobilizines are not complement-dependent. Several authors (449, 450, 598, 697) believed the test for immobilizines to be valuable. Alline and Marx (12) saw good results, principally after absorption of the sera with Reiter's spirochete. This considerably increased the specificity of the reaction. It is recommended that this principle be followed.

Immobilizine is tested for by mixing an equal amount of a live suspension of borreliae and absorbed serum according to the technic used in the borreliolysin reaction but without complement, to establish the proportion of the borreliae that have lost their motility under the influence of the serum.

The reaction has not yet been standardized. The incubation time is different, 10 to 30 minutes, and the test may be carried out at 37° C but also at room temperature before the proportion of the immobilized borreliae is determined under darkfield illumination. The procedure used in some laboratories varies principally according to the *Borrelia* strain and the availability of the live borreliae. We prefer 10 minutes incubation at 37° C with American *Borrelia* strains for routine diagnostic tests.

Utmost care must be exercised in performing both tests, to avoid loss of material and changes in proportion of the reactants. Needless to say, only competent laboratory personnel should handle live borreliae.

Cross-reactions

Frequent cross-reactions in the Wassermann and Kahn tests and with *Borrelia* antigens may be due to the close relationship of borreliae and other Treponemataceae, to the related antibody, principally of that of the immunoglobulin designated IgM as well as the affinity of the antibody for cardiolipin as pointed out by Amiraian and Leikhim (14). Positive Wassermann reactions were encountered in relapsing fever by Chang (154) in 30% of the specimens from relapsing fever patients, and often by others (263, 296, 604). The test may be positive for a transient period only (745). Positive Kahn tests were reported in 15% of the examined relapsing fever sera in China (154), and in Cyprus, for a transient period (154, 242), in some instances of *B. duttonii* infections, but Garnham *et al.* (296) recorded only negative results with the Kahn test in their patients. Others (173, 512) also pointed out the occurrence of positive results in serologic tests for the diagnosis of syphilis in relapsing fever.

No explanation has yet been offered for the positive agglutination test results with *Proteus OX* strains in some instances of relapsing fever. This cross-reaction may present serious problems when both louse-borne typhus and relaping fever epidemics break out simultaneously.

The aggultinin titer with *Proteus OXK* was reported to be frequently high in China (606), in Abyssinia (608), and in other parts of Africa (256). Positive tests with *Proteus OX19* as well as with *Proteus OXK* antigens have been recorded (395, 745). Rising *Proteus OX* agglutinin titers were observed during the course of relapsing fever, as well as positive complement fixation tests with *Rickettsia prowazeki* antigen (395).

Unfortunately, pre-infection sera are not available from patients showing such reactions. The collection of post-convalescent blood samples may also cause considerable difficulties. Further investigation of this problem is, therefore, also necessary within the huge problem-complex of borreliosis.

Differential Diagnosis

The principal differential diagnostic problem is malaria in regions where both diseases occur (11, 112). In addition to blood films and the inoculation of mice, clinical observation may be helpful. The heart and the peripheral circulation are usually little disturbed in malaria, but in relapsing fever low blood pressure and signs of cardiac failure may be impressive during the crisis. The liver is not usually painful in malaria, but it is often sensitive to pressure in relapsing fever. The headache in malaria is frontal but it is frequently occipital in relapsing fever (112). Sweating sets in early in malaria, late in relapsing fever (590).

When malaria and relapsing fever develop simultaneously in an individual, splenic enlargement and irregular fever are the outstanding symptoms (467).

Additional differential diagnostic problems are leptospirosis, plague, pneumonia, dengue fever, yellow fever, influenza, typhus, early and hemorrhagic smallpox, meningococcal infections, rat bite fever, and acute abdominal conditions, such as appendicitis, cholecystitis, peritonitis etc. because palpation and pressure often cause pain in various regions of the abdomen (690).

During World War II, the German Army on the Eastern Front was infected with louse-borne relapsing fever. Since neurologic symptoms often prevailed, the disease was mistakenly considered a new entity and named "febris neuralgica periodica" (101).

Numerous attempts have been made to differentiate louse-borne and tick-borne relapsing fever by clinical examination and observation only (186, 187), but this is sometimes an impossible task without the aid of laboratory study of the organism involved, and up-to-date epidemiologic information.

Treatment

Anti-Borrelial Agents

Arsenicals have been used in the treatment of relapsing fever practically ever since their introduction in the therapy of syphilis. Pentavalent arsenicals have been superseded by antibiotics, principally because of fewer side effects (590), and their greater efficacy.

Several investigators (154, 298, 731, 734), however, reported favorable results with arsenicals in mass-treatment during epidemics but called attention to the rather frequent Jarisch-Herxheimer type reactions that occur during the application of highly effective arsenicals.

The drug of choice of this writer (O.F.) was oxophenarsine hydrochloride (2-amino 4-arsenophenol hydrochloride, Mapharsen, Mapharsal, Fontarsan), 30 to 60 mg intravenously, preferably administered during the interval between relapses, or when the fever was rising.

The Jarisch-Herxheimer response will be discussed later because it also follows other types of treatment.

Sulfonamides have been found ineffective (380).

Antibiotics have been tested extensively in animals. Such experiments were reviewed by Vetrogradova (704) and Ercoli *et al.* (258). Penicillin was found satisfactory in the laboratory in doses of 500 to 1,000 U per Kg in rats (210, 259, 330, 412).

Penicillin in doses of 1 million units prevented relapses in human louse-borne disease (378) and was considered a satisfactory drug (323, 674). It was emphasized (443) that at least 500,000 units must be administered. Penicillin failed to prevent relapses in tick-borne relapsing fever (303, 420, 517).

Combinations of streptomycin and penicillin were found effective in rats without brain involvement by Levaditi and Vaisman (447) but were considered of lesser value by Bijlmer (77). Streptomycin, 1 Gm per day alone, did not prevent relapses in man in the Kashmir (516), nor in *B. duttonii* infections (447).

No synergism between penicillin and arsenicals was observed

(147). Neither were penicillin and chloramphenicol combinations effective in rats infected with drug-resistant *B. duttonii.*

Chloramphenicol (Chloromycetin®) was considered ineffective in *B. duttonii* infections (303). Cambournac *et al.* (140), Hirschboeck (336), and Gimeno de Sande (317) observed that 1 to 2 Gm, divided over a period of one or two days, were curative but Jarisch-Herxheimer-type reactions were difficult to manage especially in children, if such consequences of the treatment developed. The blood dyscrasias that develop during the crisis or before it may play a role in these difficulties. Nevertheless, it appears that chloramphenicol deserves further trials in louse-borne relapsing fever in adults without neurologic symptoms and without severe hematological changes.

Chlortetracycline (Aureomycin®) gave good results in rats (7, 339) but did not prevent delayed brain invasion by borreliae (351, 366). In tick-borne relapsing fever, chlortetracycline, in doses of 2 Gm per day for 7 to 10 days, was effective in trials in Eritrea (432). Satisfactory results were recorded in tick-borne infections (140, 162).

Oxytetracycline (Terramycin®) cleared animals inoculated with *B. duttonii* (75). Success with this drug was reported also in man (140, 162, 352).

Tetracycline (Achromycin®) has become the drug of choice (127, 238, 553, 562, 629). It has been reported able to clear the central nervous system of borreliae and to reduce the relapse rate. The originally recommended treatment schedule was first 0.2 Gm, then 0.5 Gm for one or two days, to a total of 4 Gm in 3 to 4 days; later 0.5 Gm every 6 hours for 6 to 7 days, or 0.25 Gm weekly to reduce the chance of relapses.

Bryceson *et al.* (127) prefer intravenous instead of oral administration of tetracycline because their patients often suffer from vomiting. One-quarter of a Gm is injected, over a period of 2 to 3 minutes. Borreliae disappear from the blood within 2½ hours. The administration of 0.15 Gm in 6-hour intervals has also been helpful. Bryceson *et al.* administer 4.5 to 5.5 Gm per os over 4 to 5 days but they have observed no relapses after a single injection of 0.25 Gm, without additional tetracycline administration.

A careful approach to therapy is indicated because possible unfavorable reactions to the treatment are not infrequent, principally when a potent drug is administered late in the disease. Parry *et al.* (562), Schofield *et al.* (629), and Bryceson *et al.* (127) described sudden rise in temperature, increase in pulse and respiration, and subjective discomfort after tetracycline administration in some patients. After the first phase of the reaction, the temperature usually decreases by lysis. This is accompanied by a fall of the blood pressure, and a decline in the number of white blood cells. These authors studied the hemodynamic and allied changes in great detail. The reaction appears to be biphasic, which led this group of investigators to the interesting conclusion that it may be due to the liberation of endogenous toxin from leukocytes. Similar reactions have been observed after the administration of other antibiotics (631) and convalescent serum (65).

In epidemics, when careful individual attention cannot be given to every patient, Bryceson *et al.* (127) have proposed the use of 300,000 U procaine-penicillin intramuscularly, and then on the next day to give orally 0.25 Gm tetracycline. Procaine-penicillin, 80,000 units intramuscularly every 6 hours in 1¼ days has been recommended by these authors when development of a Jarisch-Herxheimer reaction is feared.

Data on other antibiotics and comparison of various drugs have been published by several writers (266, 267, 631, 709 and others).

Convalescent serum, 20 ml intravenously, has been of little value to Adler and Ashbel (3) but was considered helpful by Balteanu *et al.* (65), Gaud and Morgan (298), and Sergent (639). Jarisch-Herxheimer type reactions were frequent. Moreover, "safe" convalescent serum (free from infectious agents, especially of viral and rickettsial nature) is seldom available during epidemics.

Jarisch-Herxhemier Reaction

One of the most unpleasant side effects of medication with arsenicals used to be the Jarisch-Herxheimer reaction, principally in diseases caused by Treponemataceae. Whereas in syphilis or pinta, where the number of organisms is relatively small, the sudden disintegration of the treponemas did not cause serious disturbances as a rule, being only a short exacerbation of the cutaneous symptoms with transient fever, the Jarisch-Herxheimer reaction has been a serious complication of the administration of arsenicals in borreliosis. This is due to the fact that large numbers of borreliae disintegrate simultaneously and suddenly. Originally believed to be due to liberated toxin, Parry *et al.* (1967) and Schofield *et al.* (1968) showed that the Jarisch-Herxheimer reaction in relapsing fever after tetracycline administration is allied with ventilation and hemodynamic changes different from those caused by endotoxins. The oxygen intake is increased. Arterial blood bicarbonate decreases as a result of impaired pulmonary gas exchange. Blood lactic acid is increased. The cardiac output remains high, indicating hypotension resulting from low systemic vascular resistance, at the same time pulmonary arterial pressure is increased. The administration of pure oxygen does not alter the changes in ventilation and circulation but favorably influences lactic acidosis. This may be a sign of tissue hypoxia. The lack of a favorable effect of hydrocortisone that acts as a stabilizer is also of interest. During recovery from the reaction, the mean pressure in the brachial artery remains low but cardiac output is still increased. Thus the study of the Jarisch-Herxheimer reaction in relapsing fever is unfolding new concepts of this syndrome.

Supportive Therapy

Bed rest is recommended. Sponging with cool (not hot) water is helpful.

It is necessary to restore the fluid and electrolyte balance of the patient, if it is disturbed. The venous blood pressure should serve as an indicator, as well as blood chemistry. Adrenergic vasopressor drugs must be used cautiously, to prevent diminished heat unloading during the high fever because of the vasoconstriction of the dermal vessels induced by such pharmaceuticals (127).

Schofield *et al.* (629) did not observe favorable results using hydrocortisone after the Jarisch-Herxheimer reaction developed but are in favor of administering 20 mg per Kg body weight 4 hours before tetracycline treatment.

It is customary to give vitamin K against bleeding. The usual dose is 20 mg intramuscularly.

Symptomatic treatment is often indicated, and should follow the general rules of the therapeutic indications and contraindications for the selected procedures. For instance, nausea and vomiting may require the administration of dimenhydrinate (Dramamine), 50 mg intramuscularly. Intensive pain may be alleviated by analgesics.

Prevention

Vaccines and Drugs

Aristowsky and Wainstein (25) experimented with a vaccination method consisting of injecting the blood of infected animals previously heated at 60° C for 30 minutes. It protected only against the homologous strain. Russell (619) was able to prevent *Borrelia* infections in rats by administering killed organisms together with immune serum. Sergent (639), using *B. hispanica,* could evoke premunition lasting two years with freeze-killed organisms and with bile vaccine.

Nevertheless, vaccines against borreliae for human use are not yet available. The serologic differences of the strains and their phase variations during relapses militate against the development of an effective immunizing agent.

In Tanzania, Geigy (303) observed laborers from Rwanda who carried *O. moubata* with them and permitted these ticks to feed on them periodically so as to preserve their immunity to relapsing fever. However, this method is not quite applicable to other population groups.

Drug prophylaxis trials with an antibiotic have not yet been reported but they could be considered on a theoretical basis for persons exposed to the infection for a short time only.

General Measures

Disinfection of clothing with the aid of dry heat in "delousing stations", cutting hair short, and shaving the body have been time-honored measures to prevent the multiplication and survival of lice. In addition to these procedures, Hunter (377) in Serbia during the First World War stopped railway traffic and reduced the movement of the populace to a minimum, as a general measure to halt the spread of *Borrelia*-bearing lice.

The Administration in South Africa forbade indigenous people to carry their bundles into tick-free houses, and recommended the building of cement resthouses for travelers.

Some general measures were used in the Indian Army after World War I (717). These consisted of washing or bathing twice daily, spreading the clothing on the hot sand in the sun; then taking it to a different place to be shaken out; posting guard against villagers so as to avoid contact with the organisms or their vectors; getting close haircuts if the caste permitted it; keeping out of huts and caves but staying under canvas; and turning the tents inside out during the day. This procedure was an effective preventive measure.

In Africa, the following measures were recommended (467): avoiding huts, especially those with earthen and cow dung floors; keeping out of camp sites previously used by the local population; searching lodgings for ticks; inspecting blankets of the soldiers for *Ornithodoros;* and offering a small award (one penny or so) to local children for each tick collected.

Vector Control

Dry heat and a number of chemicals kill arthropods (see above) but they withstand home illumination and ultraviolet light (364, 414).

Vectors of *Borrelia* are sensitive to DDT* dusting powder, 5 to 10%, that has proved effective against lice (251, 296). It is applied to the clothing. About 40 to 50 Gm of the powder are required for each person. Bed linen and clothing can be impregnated with a 1% DDT emulsion, using 6 volumes of emulsion for each volume of linen or clothing. In certain areas, however, lice have become resistant to DDT (135). Other dusting powders have also been considered, but 0.5 to 1% of the gamma isomer of benzene hexachloride (Gammexane®, BHC) is frequently recommended as well as 1% lindane dust. Diazonium polychlorides appear effective. Pyrethrum is used as a 0.25% powder. The effect of these contact insecticides lasts from one to several weeks.

Progress in methods used to exterminate tick vectors has been summarized by Walters (709) and Arthur (26, 27). One single spray of 3% BHC in diesoline, 600 mg per sq. ft., kept huts and coffee shops free from *Ornithodoros* for 27 months in East Africa (16). A 5% mixture of BHC in sawdust, laid in 4-inch wide bands around the base and doorwalls of the huts, kept ticks away for

*Some governments are discouraging the general use of DDT.

3 months. Tesdale (677) observed similar results. Annecke and Quinn (19) employed a 17% emulsion of 4% BHC. Less effective is the frequently used 1% dust, about 10 Kg per 100 sq. m. Holmes (370) was satisfied with 40% wettable cattle dipping powder with 5% BHC. In urban Somaliland, residual sprays of BHC, 15 mg per sq. ft., in two applications 4 to 6 months apart, were effective (461).

Pospelova-Shtrom (587) reported favorable results in Central Asia with applications of 2 Gm BHC per sq. m. in houses, and 6 to 8 Gm per sq. m. in sheds, approximately every 6 months, for 2 years. The timing of the spraying should coincide with the hatching of developmental forms of *Ornithodoros* and with the first appearance of ticks in the spring. She also stated that larvae and early nymphs are susceptible to DDT which may be used in antimalarial campaigns in the same area.

Jepson (385) recommended BHC against *O. moubata* and reported that 80 to 100% were killed in 8 to 10 days after 0.5% dust had been used. In surviving females, the eggs did not hatch. In his experience, 5% DDT powder also destroyed 50 to 80% of the ticks in about 50 days. Approximately 3 to 4 lbs were used for each 1,000 sq. ft. The floors of the huts and camps were dusted, as were a few inches of the bottoms of the walls. Re-treatment was needed every 9 months. To reduce costs, Jepson used 2.5% commercial Gammexane dust and diluted it with locally available diatomaceous earth. The final cost was about 4¼ cents per lb.

Fendall and Grounds (269) and Tesdale (678) were satisfied with the long-range effect of residual BHC application against *Ornithodoros*.

The tarring of wood cabins has been recommended to repel ticks. Leaving lights on during the night might deter any *Ornithodoros* with nocturnal habits.

Attempts to reduce the tick population by biological means are being made on an experimental scale.

Teravskii (679) studied *O. tholozani*. The ticks were exposed to 10,000 r from a ^{60}Co source that did not kill adults or nymphs of the F_3 and F_4 generations. Two thousand r, however, were lethal for larvae and the first nymphs. The irradiated adult females did not lay viable eggs. Galun *et al.* (289) studied the relationship of sexual competition in irradiated *O. tholozani* males. After 2,000 r, the males were not competitive, because of the lack of sperm. Females were sterilized with as little as 100 r. A 99% genetic lethal result could be induced by radiation, after adding sterile individuals to nonsterile tick populations. This method of insect control, particularly using competitive sterile males, was effective in reducing the tick population in caves.

Tick extermination is not practical in sparsely inhabited areas. An insect repellent is recommended for use of those who enter caves or abandoned huts, or who work around animal burrows. Dimethyl phthalate, copper oleate, benzyl benzoate, dibutyl phthalate, and diethyl lauramide have been recommended for impregnation of the clothing. Dimethyl phthalate has been extensively tested. It is often used in 5% concentration in a 2% oil emulsion. Washing with 10% carbol soap is also effective.

National and International Measures

Measures taken against relapsing fever vary from country to country. It is generally conceded that little can be done to prevent tick-borne *Borrelia* infections outside human habitations except by the use of repellents.

International Sanitary Regulations (379) require notification of cases of louse-borne relapsing fever and direct disinsection of persons arriving from infected areas before they are permitted to enter into international travel. The requirement that a passenger be free of such ectoparasites is a general health and esthetic demand. On the other hand, persons with bad hygienic habits, principally in dry and cold areas, usually move from one place to another as migrants and often cross borders illegally or without the benefit of medical inspection and examination. Despite all this, louse-borne relapsing fever has not spread in the recent past except in the Sudan and when large movements of destitute populations, dislocated by war, famine, floods, earthquakes, and other disasters, have been coupled with crowding and lack of personal hygiene. It seems obvious that surveillance of areas where migrating tribes or other groups of people move about and of neighboring territories where they visit or settle might offer better insurance against the development of relapsing fever epidemics than the international measures alone that are presently recommended. Improvement of personal hygienic practices as a result of properly conducted public health education may yield far-reaching benefits. Naturally, good results cannot be achieved through the limited medical means available to a stricken country during a national disaster, nor can the endemic focus in Abyssinia be eradicated with ease.

The problem of tick-borne relapsing fever as a disease in which animals play a role is not sufficiently emphasized in most texts. Admittedly, mammals play a limited role in the maintenance of several tick-borne borreliae. Nevertheless the habits of some ticks of associating with domestic animals is widespread and deserves more extensive study, particularly in areas where *Ornithodoros* is becoming domesticated or where it is attracted by horses, camels, cows, sheep, goats, pigs, dogs, and other animals that are in contact with man.

The story of the spreading of *O. tholozani* with camels and sheep, and the recent observations in Texas and Mexico of at least two species of *Ornithodoros* that have become domesticated show that more life science researchers, including veterinarians, must be allerted to the possibility that relapsing fever-carrying ticks are in their area, and such researchers should be encouraged to cooperate in the eradication of tick-borne relapsing fever. It could also be expected that if hunters, soldiers, vacationers, and other persons who enter tick-infested areas are educated to the possibilities of *Ornithodoros*-borne relapsing fever, this could help to reduce the number of such infections.

II

BORRELIOSIS IN DOMESTIC ANIMALS

BORRELIA THEILERI

BORRELIA THEILERI Lavern 1903 was isolated by Theiler in South Africa in 1902 from cattle with a mild disease called tick spirochetosis (681). The illness resembled piroplasmosis (cattle tick fever). There were one or two attacks of fever, loss of appetite and weight, weakness, and anemia, but hematuria was rare. A similar disease was seen in sheep and horses. The causative agent, however, appeared to be the same in all three species of domestic animals.

B. theileri is a slender *Borrelia,* 20 to 30 μ long, 0.2 to 0.3 μ wide, with 5 to 10 spirals, showing flexuous motion under the microscope. Smaller forms were seen in horses.

This *Borrelia* is transmitted by the African cattle tick *Rhipicephalus (decoloratus) evertsi.*

A similar disease in cattle was described recently in Australia by Callow (138). The *Borrelia* was 6 to 19 μ long, with 3 to 7 large, wavy spirals, resembling the smaller form of *B. theileri* from African horses. The infection was transmitted by nymphs of *Boophilus micropus,* an Australian cattle tick.

The mildness of the disease does not require treatment but tetracycline, 2 mg per Kg weight intravenously, will rid the animal of the borreliae.

Dipping cattle periodically is a measure helpful in eradicating ticks.

OTHER BORRELIAE

Borrelia hyos was described by King and Baeslack in 1913 (128). It was isolated from swine suffering from hog cholera. The organism is about 5 to 7 μ long and 1 μ wide. It can be grown in animal protein and tissue fragments containing media, but it is not the causative agent of hog cholera. Its taxonomy is doubtful.

Hjelle (367) described *Borrelia*-like organisms in the urine of lambs suffering from fever, icterus, photophobia, swollen eyelids, and facial eczema. No further data are available.

Dobell (243), Hindle (363), and others listed borreliae isolated from elephants and camels which were not studied further.

Borrelia suilla was reported by Kinmarsh in 1937 from ulcerative granulomas of pigs kept under unhygienic conditions in Australia and New Zealand. This organism should not, however, be classified with the borreliae.

III

AVIAN BORRELIOSIS

Knowles *et al.* (415), Lesbouyries (445), and Loomis (459) presented excellent reviews of this subject.

BORRELIA ANSERINA AND ITS TRANSMISSION

The causative agent, *Borrelia anserina* Sakharoff 1891, was first seen in geese by Sakharoff in Siberia. Marchoux and Salimbeni (472) established the vector and isolated the organism from fowl in Brasil. The common fowl or "blue" tick, *Argas persicus* Oken 1818, is a vector. In Brasil, *A. miniatus* was incriminated as the transmitting agent. The pigeon tick, *Argas reflexus,* is occasionally found infected with *B. anserina* in the Old World.

Argas persicus was the vector in the outbreak of "range paralysis" of fowl in Texas between 1937 and 1939 which claimed a mortality of 27 to 91% (113). Larvae and nymphs of *A. persicus* were found infectious to White Leghorns in Texas (131) and in the U.S.S.R. (540). Transovarian transmission of *B. anserina* in *A. persicus* was emphasized (361, 415, 541). The examination of the ova of *A. persicus* for small forms of borreliae is a tedious task because granules of nonmicrobial origin are present in the ova.

Nikitina (541) stated that the saliva of *A. persicus* also contains borreliae.

The red fowl mite, *Dermanyssus gallinae,* was suggested as an alternate vector. This mite remains infectious for only 3 days, and the organisms do not multiply in it according to Knowles *et al.*

(415). Hungerford and Hart (376) also conducted experiments with *D. gallinae* and were satisfied that it can transmit *B. anserina*.

Zuelzer (747) could not find *Argas* in an outbreak along the Baltic Sea and proposed that *Culex* mosquitoes are vectors of *B. anserina.* This was not confirmed by the experiments of Nieschulz and Bos (539), who observed that while mosquitoes may take up *B. anserina* the organisms disappear from the mosquitoes in a few days. Kapur (396) had the same results with *Anopheles albopictus*. McNeil *et al.* (488) and Loomis (459), studying epidemiology of infected turkeys in California, came to the conclusion that *B. anserina* was transmitted by the feces of the infected birds, or by cannibalism as reported also from India (666).

Artificially induced transmission of *B. gallinarum* by *Ornithodoros moubata* was accomplished in the laboratory (115, 284).

The blood of the chickens is highly infectious for susceptible birds.

Borrelia anserina is 6 to 30, usually 8 to 20 μ long, and 0.2 to 0.3 μ wide, with 5 to 8 spirals of various length. It is actively motile with lashing movements. It was studied under the phase and the electron microscope (229, 673) and its fibrils were observed.

The biochemistry of this *Borrelia* was investigated (385, 626, 653, 654). *B. anserina* gives the impression of being a true anaerobic organism, but does not differ from other borreliae in its enzymatic systems.

B. anserina can be stained or observed by darkfield illumination as can other borreliae. Gross and Ball (325) successfully used fluorescein-labeled antibody to demonstrate *B. anserina*.

B. anserina appears to survive in citrated blood at 0° C for 3 weeks but disintegrates in 10% saponin or bile solutions.

The organism can be cultured in Tyrode's solution or in coagulated egg white with 10% rabbit serum (288), as well as on the chorioallantoic membrane or in the allantoic cavity of developing chick embryos (91, 487).

Kligler *et al.* (413) demonstrated several serologically different types of *B. anserina*. Saurinov and Delamater (623) used agglutination and precipitation tests for the serologic differentiation of *B. anserina.* Convalescent serum kills the organisms. The borreliocidin (borreliolysin) in the convalescent serum is complement-dependent. Together with the immobilizine test the test for borreliocidin is very helpful in the diagnosis of the disease (698).*

PATHOLOGY

The organism appears to remain in the organs although only Himmelweit (359) was able to demonstrate phagocytosis of live *B. anserina*. *B. anserina* has been found in the lung, liver, spleen, kidney, and brain of infected birds but was confined to vascular and interstitial spaces. Antigen has been demonstrated in the tissues (325). Mathey and Siddle (477) studied the pathology in spontaneously infected Mongolian pheasants. There were ecchymoses under the skin, hyalin degeneration of the muscles, sometimes more extensive hemorrhages in subserosal spaces of the gizzard and the heart, eventually with necrotic foci. The spleen was small, whereas it is usually enlarged and mottled with hemorrhagic foci in turkeys afflicted with the disease. The liver is also enlarged, with hemorrhages and focal necrosis. Reddy *et al.* (601) in India found mild meningoencephalitis with perivascular infiltrates and gliosis, and necrotic foci in the kidneys as in infected chickens. The lymph nodes are often enlarged. There is catarrhal enteritis.

COURSE OF THE DISEASE

The disease caused by *B. anserina* is often called avian spirochetosis. Clinically, it begins after an incubation period of approximately 3 to 8 days, usually 4 days. The birds are cyanotic and have yellowish-greenish diarrhea, appear restless, then crouch with closed eyes. If they move, ataxia may become evident. Paralysis of the wings may be present. The body temperature reaches 43° C (109.5° F) or more in 2 to 3 days, sometimes later, and returns to 40° C (104° F) in about a week in those birds which survive the attack. The disease may last about two weeks.

Gabritschewsky in 1898 carried out a long series of experiments to demonstrate the immunologic features of avian borreliosis. Hoffman and Jackson (368) proved the identity of the disease in chickens, ducks, and turkeys. Doves, pigeons, grouse, canaries, and in

*Recently Soumrov *et al.* (Zbl. Vet. Med., *16*:328, 1969) reported excellent results with the precipitin test. Al-Hilly (Amer. J. Vet. Res., *30*:1877, 1969) recommended immunodiffusion as a practical serologic test.

the laboratory also turtledoves and sparrows acquired the infection. In some epidemics, more female than male birds become ill. Death often occurs on the 3rd or 4th day of the disease. The mortality rate may be higher in adult than in younger birds.

Young rabbits can be infected with intravenous injections of *B. anserina* but the organisms disappear in a few days. Guinea pigs, mice, rats, monkeys, and cold-blooded animals are not susceptible to *B. anserina* (86, 415, 459).

No relapses are observed. Immunity or premunition develop, lasting for several months (409) or a year (254).

B. anserina infections have been reported from Europe, Siberia, India, Africa, Australia, Indonesia, South and Central America, lately also from the Southwest and Western regions of the United States and Canada (368, 369, 399, 415, 459, 477, 718). Apparently transmission by feces of infected birds is noted more often at present than in the past.

TREATMENT AND PREVENTION

Packchanian (559) discussed chemotherapy. Penicillin is usually recommended as procaine penicillin, intramuscularly, 100,000 units. Adult chickens may be given 5,000 to 10,000 units divided in 5 to 6 doses over a period of 12 to 15 hours. Baby chicks may require much higher doses.

Diaz Ferrón (238) recommended tetracycline, 125 mg per day. In Europe, oxytetracycline, 2 mg per Kg body weight, is given in one dose, intramuscularly.

Landauer (431) recommended freshly collected blood of infected birds heated to 56° C for 30 minutes as a vaccine. Kolev (418a) in Bulgaria immunized one-year-old birds with 1 ml formolized egg-grown vaccine. Ninety-six per cent of the immunized fowl remained resistant to the disease for one year but only birds older than 4 months responded favorably.

Dickie and Barrera (239) demonstrated that after an outbreak the flock does not harbor the disease for longer than 30 days. General hygienic procedures and quarantine, coupled with antibiotic treatment, should, therefore, be successful.

IV

BORRELIAE FROM MUCOUS MEMBRANES

BORRELIAE FROM MUCOUS MEMBRANES are usually listed as *Borrelia buccalis* and *Borrelia vincentii* from the mouth and from the respiratory tract, and *Borrelia refringens* from the genitalia.

Data on these organisms are confused and meager, because the oral cavity under conditions considered normal, as well as ulcerative-necrotic lesions with low oxygen tension, may harbor organisms morphologically resembling borreliae.

Borrelia vincentii was described by Vincent in 1896 as the cause of the so-called fusospirochetal infections, among which is Vincent's angina (706). Uohara and Knapp (695) presented a review of oral lesions associated with this organism.

B. vincentii is 5 to 10 μ long, and has 3 to 8 irregular spirals. Long, filamentous forms have been observed frequently in cultures. Bladden and Hampp (79) studied the ultrastructure of this organism. It has a triple-structured wall, with cylindrical protoplasm, and intracellular concentric laminations. There are an axial filament and several fibers, usually terminating in small knobs, as well as a large number of fibrils.

Not all strains produce metabolic gas (423).

Canale-Parola *et al.* (142) described a medium for the culture of *B. vincentii*. This consists of desiccated Spirolate Broth (Baltimore Biological Laboratory) 1 Gm, desiccated Brain Heart Infusion Broth (B.B.L.) 1.66 Gm, sodium thioglycollate 22.25 mg, asparagine 25 mg, Tryptone (Difco) 25 mg, gelatin 2 Gm, and distilled water 90 ml. The pH is adjusted to 7.0. After sterilization, 10 ml inactivated rabbit serum are added.

B. vincentii is susceptible to lysis by lysozyme (518). Antigenically, it differs from other treponemes (493).

Fusiform bacilli are frequently found in lesions together with *B. vincentii.* Tunnicliff (692) suggested that they are different phases of the same organism.

B. vincentii has been isolated from acute gingivitis with painful, edematous, and ulcerated interdental papillae and marginal gingivae, from ulceronecrotic gingivostomatitis, aphthous lesions, pharyngeal ulcers and tonsils covered with strongly adherent, dirty gray membranes, peritonsillar abscess, regional lymphadenitis, and lung lesions. The disease has been designated as trench mouth, Vincent's disease, Vincent's angina, ulceronecrotic gingivostomatitis, ulceromembranous stomatitis, pseudomembranous gingivitis, fusospirochetal disease, and so on. Pain, malaise, fetid breath, bleeding, salivation, and sometimes fever with leukocytosis, shift to the left, increased blood sedimentation rate, and at times gangrene are present. When the infection is restricted to the mouth, punched-out, easily bleeding ulcers of the gums are seen. Pseudomembrane formation, noma, gangrenous laryngitis, and destruction of the gums to such an extent that the teeth fall out, as well as erosions of the bones of the oronasopharyngeal region, have been ascribed to *B. vincentii.* If the buccal mucosa is involved, more diffuse pseudomembranous lesions develop. Rectal and vaginal lesions have been reported.

The disease is more common in the undernourished, principally in children, and during wartime and other disasters (13). It has been suggested that lack of one or more vitamins may predispose to this infection.

Black (78) emphasized, however, that herpetic infections may cause acute gingivostomatitis. He investigated the oral cavity of healthy children for the presence of *B. vincentii* and found this organism in 60% of those examined. Fusiform bacilli were demonstrated in 94% of the same group, and *B. vincentii* and fusiform bacilli together in 18 to 63% of the children, according to age. It is, therefore, difficult to ascribe primary pathogenicity to *B. vincentii.*

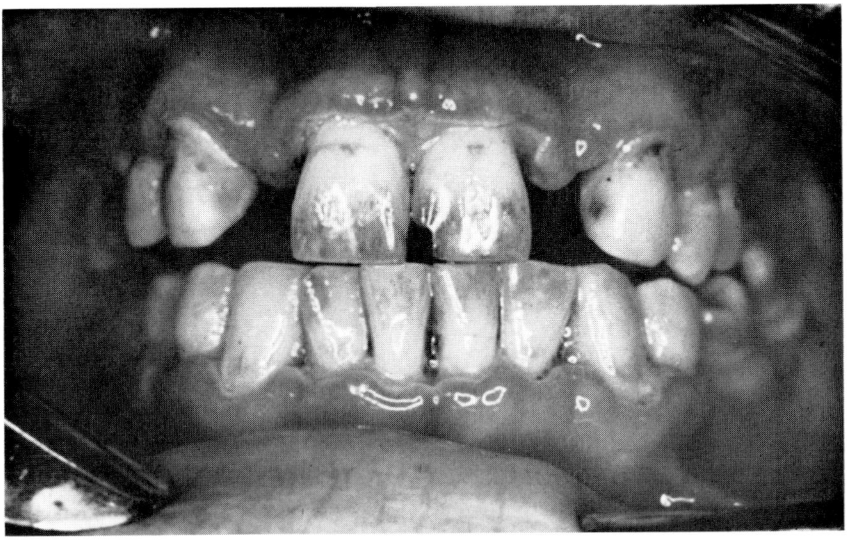

FIGURE 31. Necrotic ulcerative areas between and around the maxillary front teeth, and the central incisor region. Some necrotic and ulcerative areas also around the anterior mandibular teeth. Description and photograph by courtesy of M. N. Wilderman, D.D.S., Professor and Head, Department of Periodontology, Louisiana University School of Dentistry, New Orleans, La.

Malberger (466) in Gambia observed necrotic and ulcerative lesions of the interdental papillae in poorly nourished children with inadequate oral hygiene, with numerous *B. vincentii* present. Goldberg (319), Uohara (694), van der Veld (703), and Knox (416) reviewed "trench mouth" and acute ulcerative gingivitis. Apparently opinions concerning the pathogenic role of *B. vincentii* are divided.

The differential diagnosis must consider diphtheria, coccal infections, and malignancy.

Hydrogen peroxide, antibiotic lozenges, and zinc paste locally, and recently Metromidazole® (275) have been recommended. A mouth wash with tepid 5 to 10% sodium bicarbonate or saline is often prescribed. Vitamins C and B complex are frequently administered.

A patient with gingivitis belongs under the dentist's care.

Vincent's angina and related deeper lesions are treated either with procaine penicillin, 600,000 units daily, intramuscularly, or with tetracycline, 20 mg per Kg body weight orally, for one week.

It may be added that reports on long lasting *B. refringens* infections still appear when vulvovaginitis and balanitis are discussed in East Europe (671) but other organisms, including *Mycoplasma,* are considered the causative agents in the West.

APPENDIX

KRAJIAN'S "20 MINUTE" RAPID STAINING METHOD OF TREPONEMATACEAE IN FROZEN SECTIONS*

REAGENTS

1. Uranium nitrate . . . . 1 gm
   95% Formic acid, C.P. . . . . . . 3 ml
   Glycerin, C.P. . . . . 5 ml
   Acetone, C.P. . . . . 10 ml
   95% Ethanol . . . . 10 ml
2. 1% Silver nitrate solution, made up just before use from a 10% aqueous stock solution. The stock solution keeps for months in a dark bottle. The 1% working solution should be used the same day, not more than 3 times. Solutions with a brownish tinge are discarded.
3. Gum mastic solution.
   Saturate Absolute ethanol. . . . . . 35 ml
   with Gum mastic. . . . . 25 ml
   Let stand for 3 to 5 days in dark bottle at room temperature, shaking occasionally. Use the supernate.
4. Developer.
   Mix 40% Formaldehyde . . . . . 2.5 ml
   Acetone C.P. . . . . 2.5 ml

---

* Krajian, A.A.: *Am.J.Syph., 23*:617, 1939.

Krajan, A.A., and Gradwohl, R.B.H.: *Histopathological Technic,* 2nd ed. C.V. Mosby Co., St. Louis, Mo., 1942.

Frankel, S., and Reitman, S. (Editors): *Gradwohl's Clinical Laboratory Methods and Diagnosis,* 6th ed. C.V. Mosby Co., St. Louis, Mo., 1963.

The above is a revision by Dr. Addine G. Erskine.

Dissolve in this mixture
first Hydroquinone. . . . . 0.31 Gm
then Sodium sulfite . . . . 0.1 Gm
and Pyridine . . . . 2.5 ml
Add to above solution #3 . . . . . 2.5 ml
then Distilled water . . . . 15 ml

The developer should not be used more than 3 times. The solution will keep for 1 or 2 weeks in a dark bottle at room temperature. It should be replaced if a sediment is formed.

5. Thin celloidin solution. (Krajian formula).

PROCEDURE

a. Tissues fixed in 10% formalin at 67° C for 10 minutes are preferred. They are then frozen and sections, 7 to 10 μ thick, are washed in distilled water.

b. Prewarm solutions #1 and#4 in small Stender dishes in a paraffin oven at 60° C.

c. Prepare 3 Stender dishes with distilled water, one with about 5 to 10 ml 95% ethanol, another with 5 ml 95% ethanol to which a few drops of solution #3 have been added with a small glass lifter. (*Note*: metal instruments and tap water should not be used in this procedure).

d. Put the freshly made solution #2 in a 250 ml Pyrex or Kimex beaker.

e. Place the section in solution #1 at 56° to 60° C in the paraffin oven for 5 minutes.

f. With a glass lifter, carry it to a Stender dish with distilled water. The section should open and float. Then pass 3 times quickly but gently through the Stender dish with 95% ethanol and mastic (see under c.).

g. Rinse in distilled water in a Stender dish. The section should spread out.

h. Transfer the section to the beaker with solution #2. Heat the contents of the beaker to 70° to 73° C for 2 minutes, while exposing it to the light of a 60 W electric bulb from a distance of 4 ft.

i. Transfer the section on the glass lifter to the warm solution #4, lifting it in and out of the solution, exposing every part to the electric light and taking care that the section opens up every time it is put back into the solution. Repeat this 6 to 8 times. The tissue should appear brown.

j. Transfer to 95% ethanol to remove excess gum mastic.

k. Transfer to distilled water. If the tissue does not spread out, repeat step j for a few seconds and return section to distilled water.

l. Place the section again into the now cool solution #2 and expose to the electric light for another 10 to 30 seconds. This step is very important. Too cold or too warm silver nitrate solutions may cause improper results.

m. Transfer to a large dish with distilled water, then to a glass slide.

n. Dehydrate with isopropanol dropping it gently onto the surface of the section and leaving for about 30 seconds, blowing first gently, then harder to remove the water.

o. Blot gently with several thicknesses of Whatman No. 1 filter paper, then apply isopropanol anew to the slide for 1 minute. Drain and blot again.

p. Dip once in #5 solution. Wipe the bottom of the slide dry. Blow gently at the surface until the celloidin is dry.

v. Dehydrate in a staining dish with isopropanol for 1 minute.

r. Carry through two changes of xylene for several minutes each.

s. Clean excess celloidin around the tissue and mount in gum damar.

Treponemataceae, including borreliae, appear black against a yellow or brownish background.

This method is applicable to paraffin sections but the period of staining has to be doubled.

REFERENCES

1. Ackerman, V., and Protasov, N. (1936) Arch.Schiff.Trop.Hyg., *40*:352.
2. Addamiano, L., and Babudieri, B. (1957) C.R.Ist.Super.Sanita, *20*:440.
3. Adler, S., and Ashbel, R. (1937) Ann.Trop.Med.Parasit,. *31*:89.
4. Adler, S., and Ashbel, R. (1942) Ann.Trop.Med.Parasit., *36*:83.
5. Adler, S., Theodore, O., and Schieber, H. (1936) Lancet, *i*:448.
6. Adler, S., Theodore, O., and Schieber, H. (1937) Ann.Trop.Med.Parasit., *31*:25.
7. Adler, S., Yoeli, M., and Meerovitch, E. (1952) Trans.Roy.Soc.Trop.Med.Hyg., *46*:159.
8. Aeschlimann, A. (1958) Acta Trop., *15*:15.
9. Aeschlimann, A. (1964) Acta Trop., *21*:1.
10. Aeschlimann, A., Geigy, R., and Hecher, H. (1968) Acta Trop., *25*:176.
11. Alexandrov, Y. M. (1940) Soviet.Med., *2*:19.
12. Alline, M., and Marx, R. (1966) Ann.Inst.Pasteur *111* (Suppl.):28.
13. Alnamo, J. (1966) Sotilaslaak Aikak, *41*:73.
14. Amiraian, K., and Leikhim, E. J. (1966) Immunol., *10*:349.
15. Anastos, G. (1957) The Ticks of Ixodides of the U.S.S.R. A Review of Literature. U.S. Publ.Hlth.Svc.,Publ. No. 548.
16. Anderson, T. F. (1947) East Afr.Med.J,. *24*:259.
17. Anderson, T. R., and Zimmerman, L. E. (1955) Am.J.Pathol., *13*:1083.
18. Anduze, P. P. (1943) Bol. Entomol.Venezol., *2*:149.
19. Annecke, S., and Quinn, P. (1952) South Afr.Med.J., *26*:455.
20. Anonymus (1969) Rel.Epidem.Hebdomad.Org.Mond.Santé, *44*:425.
21. Arakhcheva, S. G. (1963) Med.Parasit.Parasit.Bolez., *32*:665.
22. Aravantinos, A. (1919) Ann.Inst.Pasteur, *33*:425.
23. Arboni, E. (1929) Boll.Ist.Sieroterap.Milan., *8*:813.
24. Aristowsky, W. M., Hoeltezer, R. R. (1929) Zbl.Bakt.Abt.I.Orig., *112*:44.
25. Aristowsky, W. M, and Wainstein, A.B. (1929), Ztschr.Immunfschg.Exp.Ther., *61*: 296.
26. Arthur, D. R. (1960) Ticks. Cambridge Univ.Press, Cambridge, England.
27. Arthur, D. R. (1962) Ticks and Disease. Row, Peterson & Co., Evanston, Ill.
28. Ashbel, R. (1942) Ann.Trop.Med.Parasit., *36*:97.
29. Ashbel, R. (1949) Trans.Roy.Soc.Trop.Med.Hyg., *42*:409.
30. Atkey, O. H. P. (1929) Bull.Offic.Internat.Hyg.Publ., *21*:1932.
31. Aubin, H., Gachkel, Z., and Gallo, M. (1947) Algérie méd., *1*:408.
32. Auboni, E. (1929) Boll.Ist.Milano Sieroterap., *8*:813.
33. Avanessov, G. A. (1938) Med.Parazit.Parazit.Bolez., *7*:88.
34. Babudieri, B. (1948) C.R.Ist.Super.Sanità, *11*:1067.
35. Babudieri, B. (1952) C.R.Ist.Super.Sanità *15*:711.
36. Babudieri, B. (1957) Bull.Wld.Hlth.Org., *16*:911.

37. Babudieri, B. (1958) Zbl.Bakt.Parasit., Abt.I.Orig., *91*:386.
38. Babudieri, B., and Bociarelli, D. (1948) J.Hyg., *46*:438.
39. Bairamova, R. A. (1958) Azerbaidzan Med.Zhurn., *11*:72.
40. Bairamova, R. A. (1963) J.Mikrobiol.Epidemiol.Immunol., *9*:83.
41. Baker, E. W., and Wharton, G. W. (1952) An Introduction to Acarology. The Macmillan Co., New York.
42. Balashov, Y. S. (1968) Parazitologiya *2*:193.
43. Ballif, L., Constantinesco, N., and Chelaresco, M. (1947) Presse Méd., *55*:586.
44. Balozet, L. (1948) Bull.Soc.Pathol.Exot., *41*:146.
45. Baltazard, D. (1936) Bull.Soc.Pathol.Exot., *29*:667.
46. Baltazard, M. (1946) Arch.Inst.Hessarak, *4*:57.
47. Baltazard, M. (1947a) Bull.Soc.Pathol.Exot., *40*:77.
48. Baltazard, M. (1947b) C.R. Acad.Sci., *225*:82.
49. Baltazard, M. (1947c) C.R.Acad.Sci., *225*:1858.
50. Baltazard, M. (1954) Ann.Parasit.Hum.Compar., *29*:13.
51. Baltazard, M., Bahmanyar, M., Habibi, A., Mofidi, C., and Seydian, B. (1950) Bull. Soc.Pathol.Exot., *43*:309.
52. Baltazard, M., Bahmanyar, M., and Mofidi, C. (1947) Ann.Inst.Pasteur, *73*:1066.
53. Baltazard, M., Bahmanyar, M., and Mofidi, C. (1948) Bull.Soc.Pathol.Exot., *41*:141.
54. Baltazard, M., Bahmanyar, M., and Mofidi, C. (1950) Bull.Soc.Pathol.Exot., *43*:595.
55. Baltazard, M., Bahmanyar, M., Pournaki, R., and Mofidi, C. 1952) Ann.Parasit. Hum.Compar., *27*:311.
56. Baltazard, M., Chamsa, M., and Chirzadi, M. (1968) Proc.8th. Congr.Trop.Med. Malar., *2*:890.
57. Baltazard, M., Chamsa, M., and Seydian, B. (1954) Bull.Soc.Pathol.Exot., *47*:878.
58. Baltazard, M., and Habibi, A. (1954) Bull.Soc.Pathol.Exot., *47*:48.
59. Baltazard, M., Mofidi, C., and Bahmanyar, M. (1947) C.R.Acad.Sci., *224*:1858.
60. Baltazard, M., Mofidi, C., and Bahmanyar, M. (1948) Bull.Soc.Pathol.Exot., *41*:399.
61. Baltazard, M., Mofidi, C., Bahmanyar, M., and Seydian, B. (1947) C.R.Acad.Sci., *225*:82.
62. Baltazard, M., Pournaki, R., and Chabaud, A. G. (1954) Bull.Soc.Pathol.Exot., *47*: 589.
63. Baltazard, M., Seydian, B., Mofidi, C. and Bahmanyar, M. (1949) Bull.Acad.Nat. Med., *133*:284.
64. Balteanu, I. (1947) Arch.Romain Pathol.Exp.Microbiol., *14*:170.
65. Balteanu, I., Russ, M. and Voiculescu, M. (1948) Arch.Romain Pathol.Exp.Microbiol., *15*:310.
66. Bannister, K. (1930) Southwest.Med., *14*:581.
67. Banwell, J. G., and Kibukamusoke, J. W. (1963) East Afr.Med.J., *20*:124.
68. Bates, L. B., Dunn, L. H., and St. John, J. H. (1921) Am.J.Trop.Med., *1*:183.
69. Beck, M. D. (1937) J.infect.Dis., *60*:64.
70. Beck, M. D. (1942) Am.Assoc.Adv.Sci.Symposium No. 18, 20.
71. Beeson, P. B. (1954) *In*: Principles of Internal Medicine, 2nd ed. Harrison, T. R. and Editorial Board, Blakiston Co., New York.
72. Belezki, W. K., and Umanskaya, R. M. (1929) Virchows Arch.Pathol.Anat.Physiol., *272*:305.
73. Bell, S. (1956) J.Trop.Med.Hyg., *59*:82.
74. Benedetto, V. di (1941) Arch.Ital.Sci.Med.Colon.Paras., *20*:168.
75. Berks, G., and Goodwin, L. G (1951) Nature, *167*:447.
76. Bianchi, C. (1947) Med.Ital., *27*:200.
77. Bijlmer, J. (1952) Antonie van Leeuwenhoek J. Microbiol.Serol., *18*:246.
78. Black, W. C. (1938) Amer.J.Dis.Child., *56*:126.
79. Bladen, H. A., and Hampp, E. G. (1964) J.Bact., *87*:1180.
80. Blanc, G.. and Bruneau, J. (1951) Bull.Soc.Pathol.Exot., *44*:313.

81. Blanc, G., and Bruneau, J. (1956) C.R.Acad.Sci., *242*:1376.
82. Blanc, G., Bruneau, J., and Chabaud, A. (1952) C.R.Acad.Sci., *234*:2577.
83. Blanc, G., Bruneau, J., and Pagés, R. (1949) Bull.Acad.Nat.Méd.Paris, *133*:600.
84. Blanc, G., and Maurice, A. (1949) Arch.Inst.Pasteur Maroc, *3*:613.
85. Blanc, G., Noury, M., and Fischer, M. (1933) Bull.Acad.Nat.Méd.Paris, *109*:587.
86. Bodechtel, G. (1930) Ztschr.Hyg.Infektkrk., *111*:348.
87. Bodman, R. I., and Stewart, I. S. (1948) Brit.Med.J., *i*:291.
88. Böger, A. (1943) Münch.Med.Woch., *90*:549.
89. Bohls, S. W. (1942) Amer.Assoc.Adv.Aci.Symposium No. 18, 125.
90. Bohls, S. W., and Irons, J. V. (1942) Amer.Assoc.Adv.Sci.Symposium No. 18, 42.
91. Bohls, S. W., Irons, J. V., and De Shazo, T. (1940) Proc.Soc.Exptl.Biol.Med., *45*:375.
92. Bohls, S. W., and Schuhardt, V. T. (1933) Texas State J.Med., *29*:188.
93. Biron, H. (1947) Ann.Inst.Pasteur, *73*:49.
94. Boiron, H. (1948) Bull.Méd.Afr.Occident.Franc., *5*:173.
95. Boiron, H. (1949a) Ann.Inst.Pasteur, *77*:620.
96. Boiron, H. (1949b) Bull.Soc.Pathol.Exot., *42*:13.
97. Boiron, H. (1949c) Bull.Soc.Pathol.Exot., *42*:62.
98. Boiron, H. (1949d) Bull.Soc.Pathol.Exot., *42*:91.
99. Boiron, H., Koerber, R., and Carronnier, B. (1948) Bull.Soc.Pathol.Exot., *41*:81.
100. Bonné, G. (1939) Ann.Soc.Belge Méd.Trop., *19*:477.
101. Bormon, F. V. (1943) Deutsch.Med.Woch., *69*:356.
102. Borrel, A. (1906) C.R.Soc.Biol., *60*:138.
103. Borrel, A., and Marchoux, E. (1905) C.R.Soc.Biol., *58*:362.
104. Bruen, F., and Blatter, C. (1960) Helv.Chim.Acta, *43*:1690.
105. Bourgain, M. (1946) Bull.Soc.Pathol.Exot., *39*:185.
106. Bourgain, M. (1947) Ann.Inst. Pasteur, *73*:84.
107. Bourgain, M. (1950a) Bull.Soc.Pathol.Exot., *43*:689.
108. Bourgain, M. (1950b) Bull.Soc.Pathol.Exot., *43*:692.
109. Bradfield, J. R. G., and Carter, D. B. (1952) Nature, *169*:944.
110. Brett, G. A. (1939) Bull.Entomol.Res., *30*:247.
111. Briggs, L. H. (1922) J.Amer.Med.Ass., *79*:941.
112. Brissolese, A. (1938) Arch.Ital.Sci.Med.Colon.Parass., *19*:377.
113. Brown, J. C., and Cross, J. C. (1941) Science, *93*:528.
114. Browse, G. V. (1912) Indian Med.Gaz., *47*:387.
115. Brumpt, E. (1908a) Bull.Soc.Pathol.Exot., *1*:577.
116. Brumpt, E. (1908a) Bull.Soc.Pathol.Exot., *1*:579 .
117. Brumpt, E. (1926) C.R.Acad.Sci., *183*:1139.
118. Brumpt, E. (1933) C.R.Soc.Biol., *113*:1369.
119. Brumpt, E. (1934) Bull.Soc.Pathol.Exot., *27*:510.
120. Brumpt, E. (1936a) Ann.Parasitol.Hum.Compar., *14*:436.
121. Brumpt, E. (1936b) Ann.Parasit.Hum.Compar., *14*:640.
122. Brumpt, E. (1937) Ann.Parasit.Hum.Compar., *15*:75.
123. Brumpt, E. (1939) C.R.Acad.Sci., *208*:2029.
124. Brumpt, E., and Brumpt, L. C. (1939) Ann.Parasit.Hum.Compar., *17*:287.
125. Brussin, A. M. (1925) Ztschr.Immun.Exptl.Ther., *44*:328.
126. Brussin, A. M., and Sternberg, E. J. (1938) Giorn.Batter.Immun., *21*:46.
127. Bryceson, A. D. M., Parry, E. H. O., Perine, L. L., Vukotich, D., Warrel, D. A., and Leithead, C. S. (1970) Quart.J.Med., *39*:129.
128. Buchanan, R. E. (Editor) (1958) Bergey's Manual of Determinative Bacteriology, 8th ed. Williams & Williams, Baltimore, Maryland.
129. Burgdorfer, W. (1951) Acta Trop., *8*:193.
130. Burgdorfer, W., and Varma, M. G. R. (1967) Ann.Rev.Entomol., *12*:347.
131. Burroughs, A. L. (1947) Science *105*:577.
132. Burrows, W. (1968) Textbook of Microbiology, 19th ed. W. B. Saunders Co., Philadelphia.

133. Buschke, A., and Kroó, H. V. (1922) Klin. Woch., *1*:2470.
134. Buxton, P. A. (1932) Biol.Rev., *7*:275.
135. Buxton, P. A. (1946) The Louse. The Williams and Wilkins Co., Baltimore, Md.
136. Calabri, O. (1959) J.Exp.Med., *110*:811.
137. Calero, C. (1946) Am.J.Trop.Med., *26*:761.
138. Callow, L. L. (1967) Brit. Veter.J., *123*:492.
139. Calwell, W. K. (1920) Lancet, *i*:785.
140. Cambournac, F. J. C., de Alemida Roque, R., and Ferreira Res, J. (1951) Clin. Contemp. (Lisabon), *5*:524.
141. Caminopetros, J., and Triantaphyllopoulos, E. (1936) Ann.Parasit.Hum.Compar., *14*:429.
142. Canale-Parola, E., Udris, Z., and Mandel, M. (1968) Arch.Mikrobiol., *63*:385.
143. Cantacuzène, J. (1920) Bull.Soc.Pathol.Exot., *13*:269.
144. Carley, J. G., and Pope, J. H. (1962) Austral.J.Exp.Biol.Med.Sci., *40*:255.
145. Carlisle, R. J. (1906) J.infect.Dis., *3*:233.
146. Carminati, G. M. (1955) Boll. Ist. Sieroterap. Milano, *34*:503.
147. Carminati, G. M. (1956) Boll.Soc.Ital.Biol.Sper., *32*:923.
148. Carminati, G. M. (1957) Boll.Ist.Sieroterap.Milano, *36*:197.
149. Casaux, J. (1912) Rev.Méd.Hyg.Trop., *9*:97.
150. Chabaud, A. (1939) Bull.Soc.Pathol.Exot., *32*:483.
151. Chagin, K. P., and Ditalov, A. G. (1960) Med. Parazit.Parazit.Bolez., *29*:288.
152. Chakrabarty, A. (1949) J.Indian Med.Assoc., *18*:352.
153. Chamsa, M. (1960) Pathol.Biol., *8*:69.
154. Chang, S. L. (1938) Chinese Med.J., *54*:163.
155. Chapcheff, C. (1925) Bull.Soc.Pathol.Exot., *18*:97.
156. Charters, A. D. (1942) Trans.Roy.Soc.Trop.Med.Hyg., *35*:271.
157. Charters, A. D. (1950) Trans.Roy.Trop.Med.Hyg., *43*:427.
158. Chen, K. C. (1941) Proc.Soc.Exp.Biol.Med., *46*:638.
159. Chen, Y. P., and Anderson, H H. (1941) Proc.Soc.Exp.Biol.Med., *46*:658.
160. Chen, Y. P., Zia, S. H., and Anderson, H. H. (1945) Amer.J.Trop.Med., *25*:115.
161. Chernyshova, T. F. (1967) Med.Parazit.Prazit.Bolez., *36*:476.
162. Cherry, J. K. T. (1955) Trans.Roy.Soc.Trop.Med.Hyg., *49*:563.
163. Chiao, S. M. (1945) Acta Brevia Sinensica, *1*:4.
164. Chiriboga, J. M. (1919) Crónica méd.Lima, *36*:127.
165. Chohan, I. S. (1966) Armed Forces Med.J.India, *22*:37.
166. Chohan, I. S. (1967) Indian J.Pathol.Bact., *10*:289.
167. Chorine, V., and Colas-Belcour, J. (1947) Bull.Soc.Pathol.Exot., *40*:383.
168. Chorine, V., and Crougue, O. (1942) Ann.Inst.Pasteur, *68*:518.
169. Chorine, V., and Crougue, O. (1943) Bull.Soc.Pathol.Exot., *36*:262.
170. Chorine, V., Grabar, P., Tixier, R., and Crougue, O. (1943) Ann.Inst.Pasteur, *69*: 162.
171. Chubaryan, Kh. A. (1966) Zhurn.Eksp.Klin.Med., *6*:39.
172. Chung, H. L. (1936) China Med.J., *50*:1723.
173. Chung, H. L. (1938a) Tenth Congr.Far East Assoc.Trop.Med.Hanoi, *2*:309.
174. Chung, H. L. (1938b) Proc.Soc.Exptl.Biol.Med., *38*:97.
175. Chung, H. L. (1938c) Trans,Roy.Soc.Trop.Med.Hyg., *31*:625.
176. Chung, H. L., and Chang, F. C. (1939) Chınese Med.J., *55*:6.
177. Chung, H. L., and Feng. L. C. (1936) Chinese Med.J., *50*:1 and 181.
178. Chung, H. L., and Feng, L. C. (1938) Chinese Med.J., Suppl., *2*:563.
179. Chung, H. L., and Wei, L. Y. (1938) Am.J.Trop.Med., *18*:661.
180. Cimino, V. (1942) Boll.Soc.Ital.Med.Ig.Trop.Sez.Eritrea, *1*:45.
181. Cimino, V. (1943) Boll.Soc.Ital.Med.Ig.Trop.Sez.Eritrea, *2*:76.
182. Clark, H. C. (1942) Amer.Assoc.Adv.Sci.Symposium No. 18, 29.
183. Closson, H. O. (1934) J.Kansas Med.Soc., *35*:53.
184. Coffey, E. M., and Eveland, W. C. (1967a) J.infect.Dis., *117*:23.

185. Coffey, E. M., and Eveland, W. C. (1967b) J.infect.Dis., *117*:29.
186. Coghill, N. F., and Gambles, R. M. (1948) Ann.Trop.Med.Parasit., *42*:113.
187. Coghill, N. F., Lawrence, J., and Ballantine, I. D. (1947) Brit.Med.J., *i*:637.
188. Colas-Belcour, J. (1960) Pathol.Biol.Sem.Hôp., *8*:73.
189. Colas-Belcour, J., Néel, R., and Vervent, G. (1952) Bull.Soc.Pathol.Exot., *45*:69.
190. Colas-Belcour, J., and Vervent, G. (1949a) Bull.Soc.Pathol.Exot., *42*:447.
191. Colas-Belcour, J., and Vervent, J. (1949b) Bull.Soc.Pathol.Exot., *42*:470.
192. Colas-Belcour, J., and Vervent, G. (1955) Bull.Soc.Pathol.Exot., *48*:747.
193. Coleman, G. E. (1934a) Amer.J.Publ.Hlth., *24*:1056.
194. Coleman, G. E. (1934b) J.infect.Dis., *54*:1.
195. Coleman, J. M., and Wright, H. E. (1942) Amer.Assoc.Adv.Sci.Symposium No. 18, 26.
196. Coles, A. C. (1936) J.Trop.Med.Hyg., *39*:77.
197. Connor, R. C. (1917) Proc.Med.Assoc.Isthmus Canal Zone, *10*:67.
198. Cook, A. R. (1904) J.Trop.Med.Hyg., *7*:24.
199. Cooley, R. A. (1942) Amer.Assoc.Adv.Aci.Symposium No. 18, 77.
200. Cooley, R. A., and Kohls, G. M. (1944) Argasidae of North America, Central America and Cuba. Notre Dame University Press, South Bend, Indiana.
201. Cooper, E. L. (1942) Med.J.Australia, *1*:635.
202. Corkill, N. L. (1948) Ann.Trop.Med.Parasit., *42*:230.
203. Correa, P., Baylet, R. J., and Parsons, L. (1964) Bull.Soc.Med.Afr.Noire Lang. Franc., 9:215.
204. Coryllos, J., and Perakis, M. (1918) Bull.Mém.Soc.Hôp.Paris, *29*:513.
205. Costiniu, J. (1920) Presse Méd., *28*:453.
206. Cragg, F. W. (1922a) Indian J.Med.Res., *10*:78.
207. Cragg, F. W. (1922b) Trans.Roy.Soc.Trop.Med.Hyg., *15*:236.
208. Culpepper, G. H (1946a) J.Econom.Entomol., *39*:472.
209. Culpepper, G. H. (1946b) J.Econom.Entomol., *39*:660.
210. Cumberland, M. C., and Turner, T. B. (1947) Amer.J.Syph., *31*:485.
211. Cunningham, J. (1925) Trans.Roy.Soc.Trop.Med.Hyg., *19*:11.
212. Cunningham, J., and Fraser, A. G. L. (1935) Indian J.Med.Res., *22*:595.
213. Cunnigham, J., Theodore, J. H., and Fraser, A. G. L. (1934) Indian J.Med.Res., *22*: 105.
214. Daels, H. (1910) Arch.Hyg., *72*:257.
215. Davidson, Sir S. (1960) Principles and Practice of Medicine, 5th ed. The Williams and Wilkins Co., Baltimore, Md.
216. Davis, G. E. (1939) Publ.Hlth.Repts., *54*:1721.
217. Davis, G. E. (1941a) Publ.Hlth.Repts., *56*:1799.
218. Davis, G. E. (1941b) Publ.Hlth.Repts., *56*:2010.
219. Davis, G. E. (1942a) Amer.Assoc.Adv.Sci.Symposium No. 18, 41.
220. Davis, G. E. (1942b) Amer.Assoc.Adv.Sci.Symposium No. 18, 67.
221. Davis, G. E. (1943) Publ.Hlth.Repts., *58*:839.
222. Davis, G. E. (1948) Ann.Rev.Microbiol., *2*:305.
223. Davis, G. E. (1952a) Exptl.Parasit., *1*:406.
224. Davis, G. E. (1952b) J.Parasit., *38*:473.
225. Davis, G. E. (1956) Am.J.Hyg., *63*:13.
226. Davis, G. E., and Burgdorfer, W. (1955) Exptl.Parasit., *4*:100.
227. Davis, G. E., and Mavros, A. J. (1955) Bull.Soc.Pathol.Exot., *48*:698.
228. Davis, G. E., and Mazzotti, L. (1953) J.Parasit., *39*:663.
229. Delameter, E. D. (1952) Trans.New York Acad.Sci., *14*:199.
230. Delanoë, P. (1929) C.R.Acad.Sci., *189*:398.
231. Delanoë, P. (1930) C.R.Acad.Sci., *191*:1481.
232. Delanoë, P. (1931) C.R.Acad.Sci., *193*:450.
233. Delanoë, P. (1933) Bull.Soc.Pathol.Exot., *26*:1249.
234. Delpy, L. P. (1949) Bull.Soc.Pathol.Exot., *42*:147.

235. Delpy, L. P., and Rafyi, A. (1939) Ann.Parasit.Hum.Compar., *17*:45.
236. Delpy, L. P., Rafyi, A., and Maghami, R. D. (1948) Bull.Soc.Pathol.Exot., *41*:136.
237. Desportes, C., and Campana, Y. (1946) Ann.Parasit.Hum.Compar., *21*:74.
238. Diaz Ferrón, E. (1957) Rev.Clin.Expañ.,*64*:97.
239. Dickie, C. W., and Barrera, J. (1964) Avian Dis., *8*:191.
240. D'Ignazio, C., and Codelconcinci, E. (1946) Boll.Soc.Ital.Med.Ig.Trop.Sez.Eritrea, *6*:237.
241. Dirk Van Peenen, P. F. (1963) East Afr.Med.J., *40*:83.
242. Dixon, K. C. (1943) J.Roy.Army Med.Corps *81*:193.
243. Dobell, C. (1912) Arch.Protistenkunde *26*:119.
244. Drake-Brockman, R. E. (1915) Trans.Roy.Soc.Trop.Med.Hyg., *8*:201.
245. Dschunkowsky, E. (1913) Deutsch.Med.Woch., *39*:419.
246. Du, S. D. (1931) Chinese Med.J., *45*:657.
247. Dubois, A. (1949) Ann.Soc.Belge Méd.Trop., *29*:15.
248. Dunn, L. H., and Clark, H. C. (1933) Amer.J.Trop.Med., *13*:201.
249. Durieux, C., and Boiron, H. (1950) Bull.Soc.Pathol.Exot., *43*:403.
250. Dutton, J. E., and Todd, J. L. (1905) Brit.Med.J., *ii*:1259.
251. Eddy, G. W. (1952) J.Econom.Entomol., *45*:1043.
252. Eidmann, E., Poespodihardjo, S., and Vinke, W. (1959) Z.Tropenmed.Parasit., *10*: 442.
253. Eisenberg, S., Gunders, A. E., and Cohen, A. M. (1968) Trans.Roy.Soc.Trop.Med. Hyg., *62*:679.
254. El Dardiry, E. H. (1945) Techn.Sci.Soc.Bull.Egypt, *243*:1.
255. El Ramly, A. H. (1946) J.Egypt.Publ.Hlth.Assoc., *21*:125.
256. Elsdon-Dew, R. (1943) Nature, *152*:565.
257. Enigk, K., and Grittner, I. (1953) Ztschr.Parasitenk., *16*:56.
258. Erocli, N., Bobalik, G., and Stubbs, R. (1956/1957) *In*: Antibiotics Annual, Medical Encyclopedia, New York, 601.
259. Ercoli, N., and Lafferty, L. C. (1944) Proc.Soc.Exptl.Biol.Med., *57*:4.
260. Falcone, G., 1951, Arch.Ital.Sci.Med.Trop.Paras., *37*:1031.
261. Favorova, L. A., Chernysheva, T F., Beshcheva, N. I., Mikhalov, A. K., and Trifonov, V. I. (1967) Med.Parazit.Parazit.Bolez., *36*:319.
262. Felsenfeld, O. (1932) Acto Med.Latina, *1*:36.
263. Felsenfeld, O. (1935) Rev.Hig.Valencia, *28*:291.
264. Felsenfeld, O. (1965) Bact.Rev., *29*:46.
265. Felsenfeld, O., Decker, W. J., Wohlhieter, J. A., and Rafyi, A. (1965) J. Immunol., *94*:805.
266. Felsenfeld, O., Volini, I. F., Ishihara, S. J., Bachman, M. C., and Young, V. M. (1950) J.Lab.Clin.Med., *35*:428.
267. Felsenfeld, O., Volini, I. F., Young, V. M., and Ishihara, S. J. (1950) Amer. J.Trop.Med., *30*:499.
268. Felsenfeld, O., and Wolf, R. W. (1969) Acta Trop. *26*:198.
269. Fendall, N. R. E., and Grounds, J. G. (1965) J.Trop.Med.Hyg., *68*:134.
270. Feng, L. C., and Chung, H. L. (1936) Chinese Med.J., *50*:1185.
271. Feng, L. C., and Chung, H. L. (1938) Acta Conventus Tertii Tropics atque Malariae Morbus, *1*:438.
272. Fenyvessy, B. v., and Scheff, G. (1930) Biochem.Ztschr., *211*:206.
273. Fisher, F. P., and Fischle, V. (1933) Biochem.Ztschr., *267*:403.
274. Fisher, W. M. (1942) Amer.Assoc.Adv.Sci.Symposium No. 18, 15.
275. Fletcher, J. P., and Plaut, C. B. (1966) Oral Surg.Oral.Med.Oral.Pathol., *22*:729.
276. Forteza Bover, J. Garriguez Orellana, A. and Marco Orts, T. (1949) Rev. Sanid.Hig.Públ., *23*:3.
277. Franchini, G. (1930) Arch.Ital.Sci.Med.Colon., *11*:449.
278. Francis, E. (1938) Pub.Hlth.Repts., *53*:2220.
279. Francis, E. (1942) Amer.Assoc.Adv.Sci.Symposium No. 18, 85.

280. Fränkel, L. (1912) Virchow's Arch.Pathol.Anat.Physiol., *18*:97.
281. Friedemann, V. (1942) Physiol.Rev., *22*:125.
282. Fry, A. G. (1920) Indian Med.Gaz., *55*:2.
283. Fuchs, P. C., and Oyama, A. A. (1969) J.Amer.Med.Assoc., *208*:690.
284. Fülleborn, F., and Mayer, M. (1908) Arch.Schiff.Trop.Hyg., *12*:31.
285. Fulton, J. D., and Smith, P. C. (1960) Biochem.J., *76*:491.
286. Gaillard, H., Lapièrre, J., and Coste, M. (1963) Ann.Parasit.Hum.Compar., *38*:1.
287. Galliard, H., Lapièrre, J., and Rousset, J. J. (1960) Pathol.Biol., *8*:77.
288. Galloway, I. A. (1925) C.R.Soc.Biol., *93*:1074.
289. Galun, R., Warburg, M., and Avidi, A. (1967) Entomol.Exp.Appl., *10*:143.
290. Galouzo, I. G. (1957) Argasid Ticks. Acad.Sci.Kazakh SSR, Alma-Ata,Translat. USNMRU #3.
291. Gambles, R. M., and Coghill, N. F. (1948) Ann.Trop.Med.Parasit., 42:288.
292. Garnham, P. C. C. (1936) East Afr.Med.J., *13*:50.
293. Garnham, P. C. C. (1947) East Afr.Med.J., *24*:47.
294. Garnham, P. C. C. (1950) Parasitol., *40*:328.
295. Garnham, P. C. C. (1958) J.Trop.Med.Hyg., *61*:92.
296. Garnham, P. C. C., Davies, C. W., Heisch, R. B., and Timms, G. L. (1947) Trans. Roy.Soc.Trop.Med.Hyg., *41*:141.
297. Gaud, M., Khalil, M. Bey, and Vaucel, M. (1947/1948) Bull.Wld.Hlth.Org., *1*:93.
298. Gaud, M., and Morgan, M. T. (1947/1948) Bull.Wld.Hlth.Org., *1*:69.
299. Gefel, A., and Rubenow, R. (1953) Harefuah, *44*:263.
300. Geigy, R. (1951) Atti 3o Congr.Intern.Ig.Med.Mediter,Palermo, 56.
301. Geigy, R. (1953a) Rev.Suisse Zool., *60*:438.
302. Geigy, R. (1953b) Schweiz.Ztschr.Pathol.Bakt., *16*:821.
303. Geigy, R. (1968) *In*: Infectious Diseases of Man and Animals, *2*:175.
304. Geigy, R., and Aeschlimann, A. (1957) Ztschr.Tropenmed.Parasit., *8*:96.
305. Geigy, R., and Aeschlimann, A. (1965) Rev.Suisse Zool., *72*.87.
306. Geigy, R., and Burgdorfer, W. (1949) Rev.Suisse Zool., *56*:334.
307. Geigy, R., and Burgdorfer, W. (1951) Acta Trop., *8*:151.
308. Geigy, R., and Herbig, A. (1955) Erreger und Überträger Tropischer Krankheiten. Verlag für Recht und Gesellschaft, Basel. Acta Trop. Suppl. 6.
309. Geigy, R., and Mooser, H. (1955) J.Trop.Med.Hyg., *58*:199.
310. Geigy, R., and Sarasin, G. (1960) Pathol.Microbiol., *24*:93.
311. Geigy, R., and Sarasin, G. (1961a) Acta Trop., *18*:359.
312. Geigy, R., and Sarasin, G. (1961b) Pathol.Mikrobiol., *24* (Suppl.):93.
313. Geigy, R., Wagner, O., and Aeschlimann, A. (1954) Acta Trop., *11*:81.
314. Geiman, Q. M. (1952) Ann.Rev.Microbiol., *6*:299.
315. Gelman, A. C. (1961) *In*: May, J. M. (Editor) Studies in Disease Ecology: Haffner Publ.Co., New York.
316. Gill, C. A. (1922) Indian J.Med.Res., *9*:747.
317. Gimeno de Sande, A. (1954) Rev.Sanid.Hig.Públ., *28*:342.
318. Ginger, C. D. (1963) Nature, *199*:159.
319. Goldberg, H. J. (1966) J.Oral Ther., *2*:451.
320. Gönnert, R., and Mudrow-Reichenaw, L. (1956) Ztschr.Tropenmed.Parasit., *7*:369.
321. Graham, M. (1931) Texas State J.Med., *27*:226.
322. Gray, J. D. A. (1929) Ann.Trop.Med.Prasit., *23*:241.
323. Greaves, F. C., Gezon, H. M., and Alston, W. F. (1945) U.S.Naval Med.Bull., *45*: 1029.
324. Greiner, J. (1921) Bull.Soc.Pathol.Exot., *14*:144.
325. Gross, W. M., and Ball, M. R. (1964) Amer.J.Veter.Res., *25*:1734.
326. Grothusen, J. (1920) Arch.Schiff.Tropenhyg., *24*:50.
327. Grün, H. (1950) Ztschr.Hyg.Infektkrk., *131*:198.
328. Guggenheim, K., Buechler-Czaczkes, E., and Halevi, S. (1951) J.infect.Dis., *89*:105.
329. Guggenheim, K., and Halevi, S. (1952) J.infect.Dis., *90*:190.

330. Guzzon, V., and Ercoli, N. (1951) Boll.Ist.Seroterap.Milano, *30*:543.
331. Haberkorn, A. (1963) Ztschr.Tropenmed.Parasit., *14*:209.
332. Haddad, C., Sheiban, A., and Budeir, R. (1946) J.Palestine Arab Med.Assoc., *2*:8.
333. Halawani, A. (1946) J.Egypt.Publ.Hlth.Asso., *21*:183.
334. Hallauer, C., and Kuhn, H. (1940) Ztschr.Hyg.Infektkrk., *122*:406.
335. Hamilton, J. B. (1943) Brit.J.Ophthalm, *27*:68.
336. Hanson, A. W., and Cannefax, G. R. (1964) J.Bact., *88*:811.
337. Harold, C. T. H. (1922) J.RoyArmyMed.Corps, *38*:398.
338. Hawkins, F. (1941) J.Trop.Med.Hyg., *44*:104.
339. Heilman, F. R. (1948) Proc.Staff Meet.Mayo Clin., *23*:569.
340. Heisch, R. B. (1947) EastAfr.Med.J., *24*:3.
341. Heisch, R. B. (1949) Brit.Med.J., *i*:17.
342. Heisch, R. B. (1950a) Ann.Trop.Med.Parasit., *44*:260.
343. Heisch, R. B. (1950b) East Afr.Med.J., *27*:1.
344. Heisch, R. B. (1952) East Afr.Med.J., *29*:327.
345. Heisch, R. B. (1953) Parasitol., *43*:133.
346. Heisch, R. B. (1955a) Trans.Roy.Soc.Trop.Med.Hyg., *49*:92.
347. Heisch, R. B. (1955b) Bull.Soc.Pathol.Exot., *48*:322.
348. Heisch, R. B., Chamsa, M., Seydian, B., and Harvey, A. E. C. (1957) Bull.Soc. Pathol.Exot., *50*:735.
349. Heisch, R. B., and Garnham, P. C. C. (1948) Parasitol., *38*:247.
350. Heisch, R. B., and Grainiger, W. E. (1950) Ann.Trop.Med.Parasit., *44*:153.
351. Heisch, R. B., and Harvey, A. E. C. (1952) East Afr.Med.J., *29*:25.
352. Heisch, R. B., and Harvey, A. E. C. (1953) Trans.Roy.Soc.Trop.Med.Hyg., *47*:239.
353. Heisch, R. B., and Harvey, A. E. C. (1962a) Parasitol., *52*:77.
354. Heisch, R. B., and Harvey, A. E. C. (1962b) East Afr. Med.J., *39*:609.
355. Heisch, R. B., Sparrow, H., and Harvey, A. E. C. (1960) Bull.Soc.Pathol.Exot., *53*: 140.
356. Hemingway, W. F., Hemingway, R. W., and Arneson, V. K. (1940) Northwest Med., *39*:362.
357. Hermant, D. (1912) Bull.Soc.Méd.Chir. Indochine, *3*:418.
358. Herms, W. B., and Wheeler, C. M. (1936) J.Parasit., *22*:276.
359. Himmelweit, F. (1933) Ztschr.Hyg.Infektkrk., *115*:710.
360. Hindemarsh, W. L. (1937) New South Wales Dept.Agric.Veter.Res.Repts., *7*:69.
361. Hindle, E. (1911) Parasitol., *4*:183.
362. Hindle, E. (1912) Proc.Cambridge Philos.Soc., *16* (part 6):457.
363. Hindle, E. (1931a) *In*: A System of Bacteriology in Relation to Medicine. Med.Res. Council.H.M.Stat.Off.London, *8*:101.
364. Hindle, E. (1931b) *In*: A System of Bacteriology in Relation to Medicine. Med.Res. Council.H.M.Stat.Off.London, *8*:147.
365. Hindle, E. (1935) Trop.Dis.Bull., *32*:309.
366. Hirschboeck, M. M. (1954) Amer.J.Trop.Med.Hyg., *3*:712.
367. Hjelle, A. (1966) Nature, *212*:856.
368. Hoffman, H. A., and Jackson, T. A. (1946) J.Amer.Veter.Assoc., *109*:481.
369. Hoffman, H A., Jackson, T. A., and Rucker, J. C. (1946) J.Amer.Veter.Assoc., *108*: 329.
370. Holmes, J. W. E. (1953) J.Roy.Sanit.Inst., *73*:262.
371. Hoogstraal, H. (1956) African Ixoidea. I. Ticks of the Sudan. U.S.NavyDept.Res. Rept.No.NM005050.20.07. Washington, D.C.
372. Horrenberger, R. (1954) Arch.Inst.Pasteur Algérie, *32*:18.
373. Horrenberger, R. (1955) Arch.Inst.Pasteur Algérie, *33*:258.
374. Horsfall, W. R. (1962) Medical Entomology. Ronald Press Co., New York.
375. Huang, V. D. (1960) Zool.Zh., *39*:595.
376. Hungerford, T. G., and Hart, L. (1938) Agric.Gaz.New South Wales, *48*:591.
377. Hunter, W. (1919) Proc.Roy.Soc.Med., *13*:129.

378. Ingraham, H. S., and Lapenta, R. G. (1946) U.S.Naval Med.Bull., *46*:1718.
379. International Sanitary Regulations (1967), 3rd.ed.Wld.Hlth.Org., Geneva, Switzerland.
380. Ishii, N., and Smimizu, S. (1941) Japan J.Exp.Med., *19*:5.
381. Ishii, N., Shimizu, S., and Tsuda, K. (1941) Japan.J.Med.Exp.Med., *19*:5.
382. Jahnel, F. (1938) Ztschr.Immunfschg., *92*:253.
383. Jancsó, N. (1918) Cbl.Bact.Abt.I.Orig., *81*:457.
384. Jellison, W. L. (1940) Pub.Hlth.Repts., *55*:206.
385. Jepson, W. F. (1947) Nature, *160*:874.
386. Johnstone, H. G. (1942) Amer.Assoc.Adv.Sci.Symposium No. 18, 35.
387. Jouveau-Dubreuhil, H. (1919) Bull.Soc.Pathol.Exot., *12*:621.
388. Jouveau-Dubreuhil, J. (1920) Bull.Soc.Pathol.Exot., *13*:38.
389. Joyeux, S., and Sautet, J. (1938) Bull.Soc.Pathol.Exot., *31*:279.
390. Juárez, N., and Fernández, S. (1954) Rev.Sanid.Hig.Públ., *28*:133.
391. Judge, D. M., and Perine, L. L. (1968) Proc. 8th Congr.Trop.Med.Malar., 894.
392. Jukes, A. M. (1912) Indian Med. Gaz., *47*:476.
393. Kalajew, A. W. (1931) Giorn.Batter., *7*:184.
394. Kalra, S. L., and Rao, K. N. A. (1951) Indian J.Med.Res., *39*:319.
395. Kamal, A. M., Anwar, M., Abdel Messih, A., and Kolta, Z. (1947) J.Egypt.Publ. Hlth.Assoc., *1*:1.
396. Kapur, H. R. (1940) Indian J.Veter.Sci.Anim.Husb., *10*:354.
397. Karwacki, L., and Krakowska, Z. (1921) Lekarz Wojskowy, *2*:27.
398. Kassirsky, J. A. (1933) Arch.Schiff.Trop.Hyg., *37*:380.
399. Kaupp, B. F. (1917) Poultry Diseases. Alexander Eger Co., Chicago, Illinois.
400. Kawamura, H. (1931) Zbl.Bakt.Parasit.Abt.I.Orig., *120*:59.
401. Kawata, T. (1957) Yonago Acta Med., *2*:142.
402. Kawata, T. (1961) Japan.J.Microbiol., *5*:203.
403. Kawata, T. and Inoue, T. (1964) Japan J.Microbiol., *8*:49.
404. Kemp, H. A., Haam, E. v., Fisher, W. M., and Evans, H. L. (1942) Amer.Assoc. Adv.Sci.Symposium No. 18, 117.
405. Kemp, H. A., Moursund, W. H., and Wright, H. E. (1934a) Amer.J.Trop.Med., *14*:159.
406. Kemp, H. A., Moursund, W. H., and Wright, H. E. (1934b) Amer.J.Trop.Med., *14*:163.
407. Kemp, H. A., Moursund, W. H., and Wright, H. E. (1934c) Amer.J.Trop.Med., *14*:479.
408. Kemp, H. A., Moursund, W. H., and Wright, H. E. (1935) Amer.J.Trop.Med., *15*:495.
409. Kervran, P. (1947) Bull.Soc.Pathol.Exot., *40*:152.
410. Kirk, R. (1938) Ann.Trop.Med.Parasit., *32*:125.
411. Kirk, R. (1939) Ann.Trop.Med.Parasit., *33*:125.
412. Kley, D., and Ercoli, N. (1950) Experientia *6*:153.
413. Kligler, I. J., Hermani, D., and Perek, M. (1938) J.Compar.Pathol.Ther., *51*:206.
414. Kligler, I. J., and Robertson, O. H. (1922) J.Exp.Med., *35*:303.
415. Knowles, R., DasGupta, B. M., and Basu, B. C. (1932) Indian J.Med.Res., *22*:1.
416. Knox, J. D. (1968) J.Roy.Coll.Gener.Pract., *16*:23.
417. Koch, R. (1905) Deutsch.Med.Woch., *31*:1865.
418. Koch, R. (1906) Klin.Woch., *43*:185.
418a. Kolev, M. (1967) Vet.Med. Nauki, *4*:97.
419. Konitzer, L. (1949) Acta Med.Orient., *8*:48.
420. Krakowski, I., and Edelstein, A. (1949) Harefuah *36*:101.
421. Kritschewski, I. L., and Dvolaitskaya-Barischewa, K. M. (1931) Zbl.Bakt.Parasit. Abt.I.Orig., *121*:421.
422. Kritschewskı, I. L., and Sinjuschima, M. N. (1931) Krankheitsforschung, *9*:139.
423. Krichevsky, M. F. and Hampp, E. G. (1966) J.Dent.Res., *45*:165.

424. Kröber, F. (1936) Arch.Schiff.Trop.Hyg., *40*:160.
425. Kroó, H. v. (1949) Ztschr.Pathol.Bact., *12*:60.
426. Krylova, D. P. (1963) Med.Parazit.Parazit.Bolez., *6*:659.
427. Kudicke, R., Feldt, A. and Collier, W. A. (1924) Ztschr.Hyg.Infektkrk., *102*:135.
428. Kudicke, R., Kudicke, H., Grammel, H. and Linhoffer, A. (1953) Ztschr.Hyg. Infektkrk., *137*:13.
429. L'Abbate, G. and Mannino, S. (1938) Arch.Ital.Sci.Med.Colon.Paras., *19*:486.
430. Lamoureaux, A. (1913) Bull.Soc.Pathol.Exot., *6*:146.
431. Landauer, E. (1931) Ann.Inst.Pasteur, *47*:667.
432. Lanzo, A., and Tresca, G. (1961) Arch.Ital.Sci.Med.Trop., *42*:434.
433. Lapierre, J., Gaillard, H., and Roussett, J. J. (1964) C.R.Soc.Biol., *158*:1047.
434. Lapierre, J., Larivière, M., and Rousset, J. J. (1958) Bull.Soc.Pathol. Exot., *51*:173.
435. Lapierre, J., Rousset, J. J., and Picot, M. (1959) C.R.Soc.Biol., *153*:1718.
436. Larivière, M., Hocquet, P., and Camerlynck, P. (1960) Bull.Soc.Méd.Afr. Noire Lang.Franc., *1*:17.
437. Leboeuf, A., and Gambier, A. (1919) Bull.Soc.Pathol.Exot., *12*:497.
438. Leeds, A. D. (1946) Parasitol., *37*:172.
439. LeGac, J. (1931) Ann.Méd.Pharm.Colon., *29*:148.
440. Legge, R. T. (1933) Calif.Western Med., *38*:370.
441. Leifson, E. (1950) J.Bact., *60*:678.
442. Leishman, W. B. (1920) Lancet, *i*:1237.
443. León, L. A., and León, B. C. (1947) Rev.Kuba *3*:145.
444. Leonova, N. A. (1945) Med.Parazit.Parazit.Bolez., *14*:79.
445. Lesbouyries, G. (1941) La Pathologie des Oiseaux. Vigot Frères, Paris.
446. Levaditi, J. C., Balouet, G., Juminer, B., and Corcos, A. (1966) Bull.Soc.Pathol. Exot., *59*:310.
447. Levaditi, C., and Henry-Eveno, J. (1953) C.R.Acad.Sci., *236*:339.
448. Levaditi, C., and Vaisman, A. (1947) C.R.Acad.Sci., *225*:769.
449. Levaditi, C., Vaisman, A., and Hamelin, A. (1952a) Ann.Inst.Pasteur, *83*:256.
450. Levaditi, C., Vaisman, A., and Hamelin, A. (1952b) Ann.Inst.Pasteur, *83*:437.
451. Levine, B. S. (1952) Publ.Hlth.Repts., *67*:253.
452. Li, Y. P. (1936) Ann.Paras.Hum.Compar., *14*:76.
453. Lipinski, W. (1949) Polski Tygod.Lek., *5*:1465.
454. Lodewyckx, A. (1938) Ann.Soc.Belge Méd.Trop., *18*:487.
455. Loewy, J. (1919) Berlin.Klin.Woch., *14*:341.
456. Lofgren, R., and Soule, M. H. (1945a) J.Bact., *50*:305.
457. Lofgren, R., and Soule, M. H. (1945b) J.Bact., *50*:679.
458. Longanecker, D. S. (1951) Am.J.Trop.Med., *31*:373.
459. Loomis, E. C. (1953) Amer.J.Veter.Res., *14*:612.
460. López Portillo, S. (1942) Rev.Inst.Salubr.Enferm.Trop., *3*:41.
461. Lovett, W. C. D. (1956) Trans.Roy.Soc.Trop.Med.Hyg., *50*:157.
462. Mackie, F. P. (1920) Brit.Med.J., *1*:380.
463. Maestrone, G. (1964) Nature, *197*:409.
464. Magee, G. R. (1942) Amer.Assoc.Adv.Sci.Symposium No. 18, 106.
465. Mailloux, M. (1962) Arch.Inst.Pasteur Algerie, *40*:344.
466. Malberger, E. (1967) J.Periodont.Res., *2*:154.
467. Manson, J. K., and Thornton, L. H. D. (1919) J.Roy.Army Med.Corps., *33*:97.
468. Manteufel, P., and Dressler, I. (1933) Zbl.Bakt.Abt.I.Orig., *130*:188.
469. Marques, A. (1943) Ann.Inst.Med.Trop.Lisbon, *1*:187.
470. Martinez Báez, M., and Villasana, H. (1945) Rev.Inst.Salubr.Enferm.Trop., *6*:185.
471. Martini, E., and Rimpau, W. (1952) *In*:Rodenwalt, E.: Weltseuchensatlas.Falk Verlag, Hamburg.
472. Marchoux, E., and Salimbeni, A. (1903) Ann.Inst.Pasteur *17*:569.
473. Margolis, A. (1919) Beitr.Klin.Infektkrk., *7*:254.
474. Marinkelle, C. J., and Grose, E. S. (1968) Nature, *218*:487.

475. Maruashvilli, G. M. (1945) Med.Parazit.Parazit.Bolez., *14*:24.
476. Más de Ayala, I. (1931) Méd.Paises Cálidos, *4*:369.
477. Mathey, W. J. Jr., and Siddle, P. J. (1955) J.Amer.Veter.Med.Assoc., *86*:122.
478. Mathis, C. (1931) Bull.Acad.Méd.Paris, *106*:188.
479. Mathis, C., and Durieux, C. (1931) Bull.Soc.Pathol.Exot., *24*:150.
480. Mathis, C., Durieux, C., and Advier, M. (1933) Bull.Soc.Pathol.Exot., *26*:1094.
481. Mathis, C., and Durieux, C. (1934) Bull.Acad.Méd.Paris, *111*:528.
482. Mayer, A. (1922) Ztschr.Klin.Med., *90*:141.
483. Mazzotti, L. (1942a) Rev.Inst.Salubr.Enferm.Trop., *3*:213.
484. Mazzotti, L. (1942b) Rev.Inst.Salubr.Enferm.Trop., *3*:297.
485. Mazzotti, L. (1943) Amer.J.Hyg., *38*:203.
486. McKee, R. W., and Geiman, Q. M. (1950) Feder.Proc., *9*:201.
487. McKercher, D. G. (1950) J.Bact., *59*:446.
488. McNeil, E., Hinshaw, W. R., and Kissling, R. E. (1948) J.Bact., *57*:191.
489. Meador, C. N. (1915) Colorado Med., *12*:365.
490. Meleney, H. E. (1928) J.Exp.Med., *48*:65.
491. Merliss, R. (1952) Med.Arts Sci., *6*:44.
492. Mersekey, C. (1947) Clin.Proc.Cape Town, 6:113.
493. Meyer, P. A., and Hunter, E. F. (1967) J.Bact., *39*:784.
494. Miller, P. B. M. (1874/1875) Pacific Med.Surg.J., *17*:370.
495. Millous, J. (1913) Bull.Soc.Méd.Chir.Indochine, *4*:14.
496. Mishchenko, N. K. (1960) Zool.Zh., *39*:424.
497. Moise, R. M. R. (1938) Ann.Med.Naval Colon., *44*:315.
498. Mölbert, E. (1956) Ztschr.Hyg.Infektkrk., *142*:203.
499. Mooser, H. (1958a) Ztschr.Tropenmed.Parasit., *9*:93.
500. Mooser, H. 1958b) Ergebn.Mikrobiol., *31*:184.
501. Mooser, H. (1963) Acta Trop., *20*:369.
502. Mooser, H., and Weyer, F. (1954) Ztschr.Tropenmed.Parasit., *5*:28.
503. Moreno Berdugo, J., and Infante Gómez, A. (1945) Med.Colon., *6*:336.
504. Moroder, J. (1929) Arch.Schiff.Trop.Hyg., *33*:603.
505. Morrison, S. K., and Parsons, L. (1941) J.Amer.Med.Assoc., *116*:220.
506. Moskwin, I. A. (1929) Ztschr.Parasit., *2*:73.
507. Moursund, W. H. (1942) Amer.Assoc.Adv.Sci.Symposium No. 18, 1.
508. Mouzels, P., and Xuang Mai, N. (1912) Bull.Sci.Méd.Chir.Indochine, *3*:427.
509. Mühlens, P. (1933) Chinese Med.J., *47*:1384.
510. Muñoz Cosin, F. (1953) Med.Colon., *22*:457.
511. Muñoz Cosin, F. (1960) Med.Trop., *35*:173.
512. Murrell, T. W. (1939) Arch.Dermatol.Syphil., *39*:667.
513. Nagano, L. (1941) Tokyo Igakai Zasshi, *3*:21.
514. Nájera Angulo, L. (1943) Bol.Réal Soc.Españ.Hist.Natur., *41*:527.
515. Nájera Angulo, L. (1945) Bol.Réal Soc.Españ.Hist.Natur., *43*:217.
516. Narain, S., and Kalra, S. L. (1950) Indian Med.Gaz., *85*:87.
517. Néel, R., Payet, M., and Gonnet, C. (1949) Bull.Soc.Pathol.Exot., *42*:384.
518. Nevin, T. A., and Guest, W. J. (1967) J.Bact., *94*:1388.
519. Newcomb, C. (1920) Indian Med.Gaz., *55*:208.
520. Nicolle, C., and Anderson, C. (1926) Arch.Inst.Pasteur Tunis, *15*:197.
521. Nicolle, C., and Anderson, C. (1927a)Bull.Inst.Pasteur, *25*:657.
522. Nicolle, C., and Anderson, C. (1927b) Arch.Inst.Pasteur Tunis, *16*:123.
523. Nicolle, C., and Anderson, C. (1929a) C.R.Acad.Sci., *189*:817.
524. Nicolle, C., and Anderson, C. (1929b) Acta Med.Scandin., *70*:392.
525. Nicolle, C., and Anderson, C. (1929c) Arch.Inst.Pasteur Tunis, *18*:268.
526. Nicolle, C., and Anderson, C. (1930) Arch.Inst.Pasteur Tunis, *19*:469.
527. Nicolle, C., and Anderson, C. (1932) C.R.Acad.Sci., *194*:333.
528. Nicolle, C., Anderson, C., and Colas-Belcour, J. (1929) C.R.Acad.Sci., *189*:224.
529. Nicolle, C., Anderson, C., and Colas-Belcour, J. (1930) Arch.Inst.Pasteur Tunis *19*:133.

530. Nicolle, C., Anderson, C., and Hornus, P. (1929) C.R.Acad.Sci., *188*:1211.
531. Nicolle, C., and Blaizot, L. (1912a) Bull.Soc.Pathol.Exot., *5*:472.
532. Nicolle, C., and Blaizot, L. (1912b) Arch.Inst.Pasteur Tunis, *1*:201.
533. Nicolle, C., and Blaizot, L. (1913) Bull.Soc.Pathol.Exot., *6*:107.
534. Nicolle, C., Blaizot, L., and Conseil, E. (1912a) C.R.Acad.Sci., *154*:1636.
535. Nicolle, C., Blaizot, L., and Conseil, E. (1912b) C.R.Acad.Sci., *155*:481.
536. Nicolle, C., Blaizot, L., Conseil, E. (1913) Bull.Soc.Path.Exot., *6*:106.
537. Nicolle, C., and Lebrailly, C. (1919) C.R.Acad.Sci., *169*:934.
538. Nicolle, C., and Lebrailly, C. (1920) Arch.Inst.Pasteur Tunis, *11*:131.
539. Nieschulz, O. v., and Bos, A. (1940) Zbl.Bakt.Abt.I.Orig., *145*:258.
540. Nikitina, R. E. (1965a) Sbor.Trud.Vsech.Nauch.Bolez.Ptits, *1*:164.
541. Nikitina, R. E. (1965b) Zool.Zh., *44*:294.
542. Nixon, A. (1921) Lancet, *i*:432.
543. Noble, R. E., and Noble, C. A. (1964) Parasitology, 2nd ed. Lea and Febiger, Philadelphia, Pennsylvania.
544. Noguchi, H. (1912a) J.Exp.Med., *16*:199.
545. Noguchi, H. (1912b) Münch.Med.Woch., *59*:1937.
546. Nohira, A. (1929) Japan.Med.World, *9*:83.
547. Novy, F. G., and Knapp, R. E. (1906) J.infect.Dis., *3*:291.
548. Nuttall, G. H. F. (1913) Parasitol., *5*:262.
549. Oag, R. K. (1939) J.Pathol.Bact., *49*:339.
550. Oag, R. K. (1940) J.Pathol.Bact., *51*:127.
551. Oettinger, J., and Halbreich, J. (1922) Münch.Med.Woch., *69*:778.
552. Omar, M. E. S. (1946) J.Egypt.Publ.Hlth.Assoc., *21*:195.
553. Ombati, D. G., and Ojiambo, H. P. (1968) EastAfr.Med.J., *45*:630.
554. Omori, N. (1939) Taiwan Igakai Zasshii, *38*:899.
555. Ordman, D. (1939) South Afr.Med.J., *13*:491.
556. Ordman, D. (1955) South Afr.Med.J., *29*:518.
557. Ordman, D., and Jones, F. R. (1940) South Afr.Med.J., *14*:81.
558. Osorno Mesa, S. (1942) Rev.Fac.Nac.Agronom.Medellin, *16/17*:1.
559. Packchanian, A. H. (1950) Texas Repts.Biol.Med., *8*:78.
560. Palmer, J. H., and Crawford, D. J. M. (1933) J.CanadianMed.Assoc., *28*:643.
561. Pampana, E. J. (1931) Arch.Ital.Sci.Med.Colon., *12*:257.
562. Parry, E. H. O., Bryceson, A. D. M., and Leihead, C. S. (1967) Lancet, *i*:81.
563. Pavolvskii, E. N. (1932) Trudy Soviet.Izuch.Proizvod.Turkmenia, *2*:79.
564. Pavlovskii, E. N. (1939) Prob.Region.Parasitol., *3*:19.
565. Pavlovskii, E. N. (1943) C.R.Acad.Sci.U.S.S.R., *39*:286
566. Pavlovskii, E. N. (1945) Med.Parasit.Parasit.Bolez., *14*:56.
567. Pavlovskii, E. N., and Kuzima, L. A. (1945) Med.Parazit.Parazit.Bolez., *14*:66.
568. Pavlovskii, E. N., and Skrynnik, A. N. (1945) Zool.Zh., *24*:161.
569. Pavlovskii, E. N., and Skrynnik, A N. (1951) Dokl.Akad.Nauk U.S.S.R., *78*:1069.
570. Petrilla, A., and Rudnay, O. (1949) Népegészségügy, *30*:439.
571. Petrishcheva, P. A. (1961) Med.Parazit.Parazit.Bolez., *30*:439.
572. Pfister, R. (1949) Bull.Soc.Pathol.Exot., *42*:547.
573. Pifano, F. (1941) Rev. Sanid.Asist.Soc.Caracas, *6*:787.
574. Pillot, J. (1966) Biol.Med.(Paris), *55*:343.
575. Pillot, J., Dupouey, P., and Ryter, A. (1954) Ann.Inst.Pasteur, *107*:489 and 663.
576. Pillot, J., and Ryter, A. (1965) Ann.Inst.Pasteur, *108*:791.
577. Pino-Pou, R. (1921) Gac.Méd.Caracas, *28*:111.
578. Pinto, M. R. (1945) Arq.Inst.Bacteriol. Camara Pestana, *9*:224.
579. Pirot, R., and Bourgain, M. (1945a) Bull.Soc.Pathol.Exot., *38*:12.
580. Pirot, R., and Bourgain, M. (1945b) Bull.Soc.Pathol.Exot., *38*:88.
581. Pirot, R., and Bourgain, M. (1945a) Bull.Soc.Pathol.Exot., *38*:90.
582. Plaut, F., and Steiner, G. (1920a) Arch.Schiff.Trop.Hyg., *24*:33.
583. Plaut, F., and Steiner, G. (1920b) Deutsch.Med.Woch., *46*:1101.
584. Popow, P. P., and Achundow, I. A. (1936) Arch.Schiff.Trop.Hyg., *40*:289.

585. Popow, P. P., and Achundow, I. A. (1940) Med.Parazit.Parazit.Bolez., *9*:255.
586. Pospelova-Shtrom, M. V. (1940) Med.Parazit.Parazit.Bolez., *9*:618.
587. Pospelova-Shtrom, M. V. (1968) Proc.8th Internat.Congr.Trop.Med.Malar., 888.
588. Prado, E. del (1919) Crónica Méd.Lima, *36*:408.
589. Prado, E. del (1920) Ann.Fac.Méd.Lima, *3*:26 and 134.
590. Quinn, C. E., and Perkins, E. S. (1946) J.Trop.Med.Hyg., *49*:30.
591. Rafyi, A. (1946a) Arch.Inst.Hessarek, *2*:37.
592. Rafyi, A. (1946b) Arch.Inst.Hessarek, *4*:49 and Sem. Hôp.Paris, *23*:76.
593. Rafyi, A., Felsenfeld, O., Dupont, J. R., and Maghami, G. (1965) Ann.Parasit.Hum. Compar., *40*:631.
594. Rafyi, A., and Maghami, G. R. (1949) Bull.Soc.Pathol.Exot., *42*:215.
595. Rahaman, A. H. (1946) J.Egypt.Publ.Hlth.Assoc., *21*:125.
596. Ranque, J. (1963) Transfusion (Paris), *6*:163.
597. Ranque, J. (1968) Méd.Trop.(Marseille), *27*:519.
598. Ranque, J., Depieds, R., and Fauré, A. (1957) Bull.Soc.Pathol.Exot., *50*:360.
599. Ranque, J., Quilici, M., and Assadourian, Y. (1968) Proc.8th Internat.Congr.Trop. Med.Malar., *2*:893.
600. Rao, K. N. A., and Kalra, S. L. (1949) Indian J.Med.Res., *37*:385.
601. Reddy, V. M., Ramachandran, P. K., and Ramachandran, S. (1966) Indian J.Veter. Sci.Anim.Husb., *36*:1.
602. Remlinger, P., and Bailly, J. (1929) C.R.Soc.Biol., *102*:741.
603. Riding, D., and McDowell, T. W. (1927) Trans.Roy.Soc.Trop.Med.Hyg., *20*:524.
604. Roaf, H. E. (1922) Brit.J.Exp.Pathol., *3*:59.
605. Robertson, A. (1935) J.Trop.Med.Hyg., *38*:237.
606. Robertson, R. C. (1932) Chinese Med.J., *20*:524.
607. Robinson, P. (1942) Brit.Med.J., *ii*:216.
608. Robinson, S. P. (1943) Ann.Trop.Med.Parasit., *37*:38.
609. Rodhain, J., and Bergh, L. van den (1943) Ann.Soc.Belge Méd.Trop., *23*:141.
610. Rodino, N. (1922) Giorn.Med.Milit., *70*:90.
611. Rosenholz, H. P. (1927) Cbl.Bact.Abt.I.Orig., *102*:179.
612. Ross, P. H. (1912) Nairobi Lab.Publ.Hlth.Repts., *2*(part 2):6.
613. Ross, P. H., and Milne, A. D. (1904) Brit.Med.J., *ii*:1453.
614. Roy, S. C. (1920) Indian Med.Gaz., *56*:320.
615. Rubinstein, P. L., and Kapusto, M. L. (1931) Ztschr.Immunfschg.Exp.Ther., *72*:309.
617. Russell, H. (1932) Trans.Roy.Soc.Trop.Med.Hyg., *26*:259.
618. Russel, H. (1933) West Afr.Med.J., *6*:36.
619. Russell, H. (1936) Trans.Roy.Soc.Trop.Med.Hyg., *30*:179.
620. Sabalette, R., Dominguez, M., and Iglesias, R. (1947) Med.Colon.(Madrid), *9*:207.
621. Saglam, T. (1947) Türk Tip Cemiyeti Mekmuasi, *13*:36.
622. Sarasin, G. (1959) Acta Trop., *16*:218.
623. Saurinov, V. R., and Delamater, E. D. (1952) Am.J.Syph., *36*:352.
624. Sautet, J. (1937) Marseille Méd., *74*:273.
625. Sautet, J. (1941) Arch.Inst.Pasteur Algérie, *19*:240.
626. Scheff, G. (1935) Zbl.Bakt.Parasit.Abt.I.Orig., *134*:35.
627. Scheff, G. J., and Kutner, F. R. (1959) Experientia, *15*:342.
628. Schilling, V. (1921) Beiheft.Arch.Schiff.Trop.Hyg., *25*:5.
629. Schofield, T. P. C., Talbot, J. M., Bryceson, A. D. M., and Parry, E. H. O. (1968) Lancet *ii*:58.
630. Schuhardt, V. T. (1942) Amer.Assoc.Adv.Sci.Symposium No. 18, 58.
631. Schuhardt, V. T. (1952) Ann.New York Acad.Sci., *55*:1209.
632. Schuhardt, V. T., and Wilkerson, M. (1951) J.Bact., *62*:215.
633. Schwetz, J. (1943) Ann.Soc.Belge Méd.Trop., *23*:219.
634. Scott, H. H. (1942) A History of Tropical Medicine, *2*:781. The Williams and Wilkins Co., Baltimore, Maryland.
635. Scott, R. B. (1944) Lancet, *ii*:436.

636. Selwyn-Clarge, P. S. LeFanu, G. H., and Ingram, A. (1923) Ann.Trop.Med.Parasit., *17*:389.
637. Sergent, A. (1933) C.R.Acad.Sci., *197*:717.
638. Sergent, A. (1936) C.R.Soc.Biol., *14*:1520.
639. Sergent, A. (1938) Arch.Inst.Pasteur, *61*:217.
640. Sergent, E. (1945) Ann.Inst.Pasteur Algerie, *23*:245.
640a. Sergent, E. (1957) Ztschr.Tropenmed.Parasit., *3*:242.
641. Sergent, E., and Foley, H. (1908) Bull.Soc.Pathol.Exot., *1*:174.
642. Sergent, E., and Foley, H. (1921) Bull.Soc.Pathol.Exot., *14*:632.
643. Sergent, E., and Poncet, A. (1961) Arch.Inst.Pasteur Algerie, *39*:109.
644. Serstnev, E. (1953) Higijena, *5*:106.
645. Shrimpton, E. A. G. (1936) Chinese Med.J.Suppl.I, 312.
646. Sibilia, D. (1937) Policlinico, *44*:722.
647. Simmons, J. S. (1955) *In*: Cecil, R. L.: Textbook of Medicine, 9th ed. Saunders & Co., New York.
648. Simons, H. (1939) Ann.Parasitol.Hum.Compar., *17*:62.
649. Skinner, J. E., Trimble, C. G., and Cheng, C. G. (1919) Chinese Med.J., *33*:210.
650. Skrynnik, A. N. (1968) Parazitologiia, *2*:3.
651. Slavina, N. S. (1944) Med.Parazit.Parazit.Bolez., *13*:85.
652. Smith, L., and Brown, T. G. (1969) California Med., *101*:322.
653. Smith, P. J. C. (1960a) Biochem.J., *76*:500.
654. Smith, P. J. C. (1960b) Biochem.J., *76*:508.
655. Sofiev, M. S. (1941) Med.ParazitParazit.Bolez., *10*:267.
656. Sofiev, M. S., and Leitman, M. Z. (1946) Med.Parazit.Parazit.Bolez., *15*:81.
657. Sofiev, M. S., and Leonova, N. A., (1945) Med.Parazit.Bolez., *14*:60.
658. Soule, M. H. (1942) Amer.Assoc.Adv.Sci.Symposium No. 18, 53.
659. Southern, P. M. Jr., and Sanford, J. P. (1968) Medicine, *48*:129.
660. Sparrow, H. (1955a) Arch.Inst.Pasteur Tunis, *32*:25.
661. Sparrow, H. (1955b) C.R.Acad.Sci., *241*:1636.
662. Sparrow, H. (1956a) Bull.Soc.Pathol.Exot., *49*:630.
663. Sparrow, H. (1956b) Arch.Inst.Pasteur Tunis, *33*:163.
664. Sparrow, H. (1958) Bull.Wild.Hlth.Org., *19*:673.
665. Sparrow, H. (1959) Proc.6th Internat.Congr.Trop.Med.Malar., *4*:484.
666. Sreenivasan, M. K., and Sankaranarayan, N. S. (1945) Indian Veter.J., *21*:325.
667. Stavitsky, A. B. (1948) Bact.Rev., *12*:203.
668. Stein, G. J. (1944) J.Exp.Med., *79*:115.
669. Sterling-Okunewski, S. (1919) Cbl.Bact.Abt.,I,Orig., *82*:456.
670. Stuart, G. (1945) Epidem.Inform.Bull.U.N.R.R.A., *1*:453.
671. Suchanek, J., Ciecierski, L., and Lawrynowycz, R. (1957) Polski Tygod.Lek., *22*: 1103.
672. Sudley, E. W. (1920) Bull.Soc.Pathol.Exot., *13*:63.
673. Swain, R. H. A. (1955) J.Pathol.Bact., *69*:117.
674. Taft, W. C., and Pike, J. B. (1945) J.Amer.Med.Assoc., *129*:1002.
675. Talice, R. V. (1929) Ann.Parasit.Hum.Compar., *7*:177 .
677. Tesdale, C. (1952) East Afr.Med.J., *29*:138.
678. Tesdale, C. (1965) East Afr.Med.J., *52*:529.
679. Teravskii, I. K. (1966) Zool.Zh., *45*:371.
680. Thayer, K. H. (1940) Southwest.Med., *24*:125.
681. Theiler, A. (1902) J.Compar.Pathol.Ther., *17*:47.
682.Thiel, P. H. van (1960) Acta Leidensia, *30*:123.
683. Toda, T., and Hiroki, H. (1934) Ztschr.Immunfschg.Exp.Ther., *82*:1.
684. Todd, J. L. (1913) Proc.Soc.Exp.Biol., *10*:134.
685. Todd, J. L. (1919) Bull.Soc.Pathol.Exot., *12*:1290.
686. Tongeren, H. A. E. van, and Koetsier, J. C. (1968) Nederl.Tijd.Geneesk., *112*:1778.
687. Toyoda, H. (1919) Kitsato Arch.Exp.Med., *3*:42.

688. Toyoda, H. (1920) Kitasato Arch.Exp.Med., *4*:40.
689. Trautmann, R. (1907) Ann.Inst.Pasteur, *21*:808.
690. Trimarchi, M. (1942) Boll.Soc.Ital.Med.Ig.Trop.Sez.Eritrea, *1*:93.
691. Troitskii, N. V. (1945) Med.Parazit.Parazit.Bolez., *14*:70.
692. Tunnicliff, R. (1906) J.infect.Dis., *3*:148.
693. Turner, L. H. (1968) Trans.Roy.Soc.Trop.Med.Hyg., *62*:880.
694. Uohara, G. I. (1967) Oral Surg., *24*:113.
695. Uohara, G. I., and Knapp, M. J. (1967) Oral Surg.Oral Med.Oral Pathol., *24*:113.
696. Vago, S. (1947) Wien.Med.Woch., *97*:429.
697. Vaisman, A., and Hamelin, A. (1954) Ann.Inst.Pasteur, *86*:107 .
698. Varma, K. C., and Malik, B. S. (1968) Current Sci., *37*:170.
699. Varma, M. G. R. (1956a) Ann.Trop.Med.Parasit., *50*:1.
700. Varma, M. G. R. (1956b) Ann.Trop.Med.Parasit., *50*:18.
701. Varma, M. G. R. (1956c) Trans.Roy.Soc.Trop.Med.Hyg., *50*:234.
702. Vassiliadis, P., and Jardin, J. (1930) Ann.Soc.Belge.Méd.Trop., *10*:133.
703. Veld, R. G. van der (1967) Nederl.Tijd.Tandheelk., *74*:628.
704. Vertogradova, T. P. (1957) Antibiotiki, *3*:44.
705. Vigors, E. G. K. (1944) Rev.Ecuator.Hig.Med.Trop., *1*:362.
706. Vincent, H. (1896) Ann.Inst.Pasteur, *10*:488.
707. Vincent, R. (1927) Ann.Inst.Pasteur, *41*:131.
708. Wagner-Jevseenko, O. (1958) Acta Trop., *15*:118.
709. Walters, J. H. (1961) *In*: Woodruff, A. W., and Walters, J. H.: Recent Advances in Tropical Medicine, 3rd ed. J.&H.Churchill Ltd., London
710. Walton, G. A. (1951) East Afr.Med.J., *28*:189.
711. Walton, G. A. (1953) Trans.Roy.Soc.Trop.Med.Hyg., *47*:410.
712. Walton, G. A. (1955) East Afr.Med.J., *32*:377.
713. Walton, G. A. (1957) Bull.Entomol.Res., *48*:669.
714. Walton, G. A. (1959) Proc.Roy.Soc.Entomol.London, *34*:63.
715. Walton, G. A. (1962) Symposia Roy.Zoolog.Soc.London, *6*:83.
716. Wang, C. W., and Lee, C. U. (1936) Chinese Med.J., *50*:241.
717. Wanhill, A. J. (1919) J.Roy.Army Med.Corps, *33*:178.
718. Ward, A. R., and Gallagher, B. A. (1920) Diseases of Domestic Birds. The Macmillan Co., New York.
719. Weichbrodt, R. (1921) Ztschr.Immunfschg., *33*:267.
720. Weiss, E. (1929) J.Lab.Clin.Med., *14*:1191.
721. Weitz, B., and Buxton, P. A. (1953) Bull.Entomol.Res., *44*:445.
722. Weller, B., and Graham, G. M. (1930) J.Amer.Med.Assoc., *95*:1834.
723. Westphal, A. (1963) Arch.Hyg.Bact., *147*:349.
724. Weyer, F. (1960) Ann.Rev.Entomol., *5*:405
725. Weyer, F. (1968) Ztschr.Tropenmed.Parasit., *19*:344.
726. Weyer, F., and Mooser, H. (1957) Ztschr.Tropenmed.Parasit., *8*:294.
727. Wheeler, C. M. (1938) Am.J.Trop.Med., *18*:641.
728. Wheeler, C. M. (1942) Amer.Assoc.Adv.Sci.Symposium No. 18, 89.
729. Wheeler, C. M (1943) J.Parasit., *29*:33.
730. Wheeler, C. M., Herms, W. B., and Meyer, K. F. (1935) Proc.Soc.Exptl.Biol.Med., *32*:1290.
731. Whitmore, E. R. (1930) *In*: Tice, F.: Practice of Medicine. W.F.Prior Co., Hagerstown, Md.
732. Whitmore, E. R. (1966) *In*: Tice-Harvey: Practice of Medicine, *4*. W.F.Prior Co., Hagerstown, Maryland.
733. Wilcox, C. (1944) Trop.Med.Bull., *41*:791.
734. Willcox, W. H. (1920) Proc.Roy.Soc.Med., *13*:59.
735. Wilson, G. S., and Miles, A. A. (1964) Principles of Bacteriology and Immunity, 5th ed. The Williams and Wilkins Co., Baltimore, Maryland.
736. Wolman, B., and Wolman, M. (1945) Ann.Trop.Med.Parasit., *39*:82.

737. Wolstenhome, B., and Gear, J. H. S. (1948) Trans.Roy.Soc.Trop.Med.Hyg., *41*:513.
738. Wood, R. C., and Dixon, K. C. (1945) Brit.Med.J., *ii*:526.
739. Wright, H. D., and Harold, C. H. H. (1919) J.Roy.Army.Med.Corps, *35*:203.
740. Wynns, H. L. (1942) Amer.Assoc.Adv.Sci.Symposium No. 18, 100.
741. Wynns, H. L., and Beck, M. D. (1935) Amer.J.Publ.Hlth., *25*:270.
742. Yeo, R. M. (1950) South Afr.Med.J., *24*:457.
743. Young, H. (1951) Ann.Biol.Chim., *9*:318.
744. Zaharia, N. I. (1948) Rev.Stiint.Med.Bucurest, *57*:209.
745. Zarafonetis, C. J. D., Ingham, H. S., and Berry, J. F. (1946) J.Immunol., *52*:189.
746, Zhordania-Rapava, T. K. (1958) Med.Parazit.Parazit.Bolez., *27*:397.
747. Zuelzer, M. (1936) J.Trop.Med., *39*:204.
748. Zumpt, F. (1959) Nature, *184*:793.
749. Zumpt, F., and Organ, D. (1961) South Afr.J.Lab.Clin.Med., *7*:31.

INDEX

P

R

S

X

Y